total
foam rolling
techniques

TRADE SECRETS OF A PERSONAL TRAINER

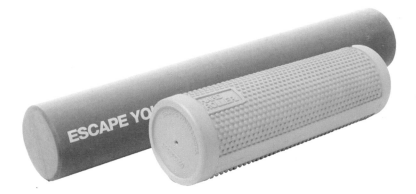

Note

Whilst every effort has been made to ensure that the content of this book is as technically accurate and as sound as possible, neither the author nor the publishers can accept responsibility for any injury or loss sustained as a result of the use of this material.

Published by Bloomsbury Publishing Plc
50 Bedford Square, London WC1B 3DP
www.bloomsbury.com

Bloomsbury is a trademark of Bloomsbury Publishing Plc

First edition 2014

Copyright © 2014 Steve Barrett

ISBN (print) 978 1 4729 0664 9
ISBN (epub): 978 1 4729 1148 3
ISBN (epdf): 978 1 4729 1149 0

Acknowledgements
Cover photographs © ESC Creative LLP: www.esccreative.com
Inside photographs © ESC Creative LLP with the exception of the following, pp. 28 and 34 © Shutterstock.com
Illustrations © Shutterstock
Designed by James Watson
Commissioned by Charlotte Croft
Edited by Sarah Cole

This book is produced using paper that is made from wood grown in managed, sustainable forests. It is natural, renewable and recyclable. The logging and manufacturing processes conform to the environmental regulations of the country of origin.

Typeset in 10.25pt on 13.5pt URWGroteskLig by Margaret Brain, Wisbech

Printed and bound in China by C & C Offset Printing Co., Ltd.

10 9 8 7 6 5 4 3 2 1

total foam rolling techniques

TRADE SECRETS OF A PERSONAL TRAINER

STEVE BARRETT

B L O O M S B U R Y

LONDON • NEW DELHI • NEW YORK • SYDNEY

disclaimer and advisory

Before attempting any form of exercise, always ensure you have a safe working environment. Ensure that the floor surface you are on is non-slip, and do not stand on any rugs or mats that could move when you exercise. Also, clear your exercise space of items that could cause you harm if you collided with them; this includes furniture, pets and children. Pay particular attention to the amount of clearance you have above your head and remember that for some of the exercise moves you will be raising your hands above head height, so keep away from doorways and light fittings.

The information, workouts, health-related information and activities described in this publication are practised and developed by the author and should be used as an adjunct to your understanding of health and fitness and, in particular, strength training. While physical exercise is widely acknowledged as being beneficial to a participant's health and well-being, the activities and methods outlined in this book may not be appropriate for everyone. It is fitness industry procedure to recommend all individuals, especially those suffering from disease or illness, to consult their doctor for advice on their suitability to follow specific types of activity. This advice also applies to any person who has experienced soft tissue or skeletal injuries in the past, those who have recently received any type of medical treatment or are taking medication and women who are, or think they may be, pregnant.

The author has personally researched and tried all of the exercises, methods and advice given in this book on himself and with many training clients. However, this does not mean these activities are universally appropriate and neither he nor the publishers are, therefore, liable or responsible for any injury, distress or harm that you consider may have resulted from following the information contained in this publication.

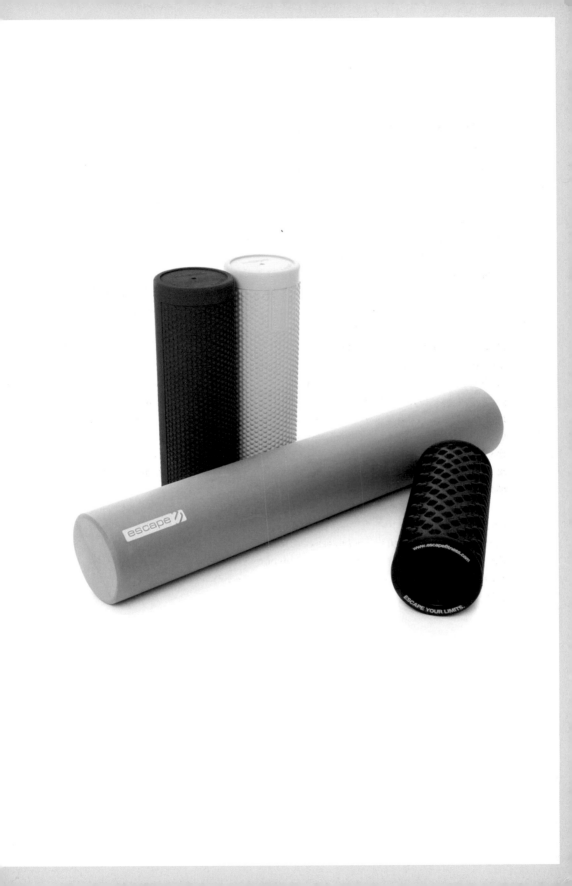

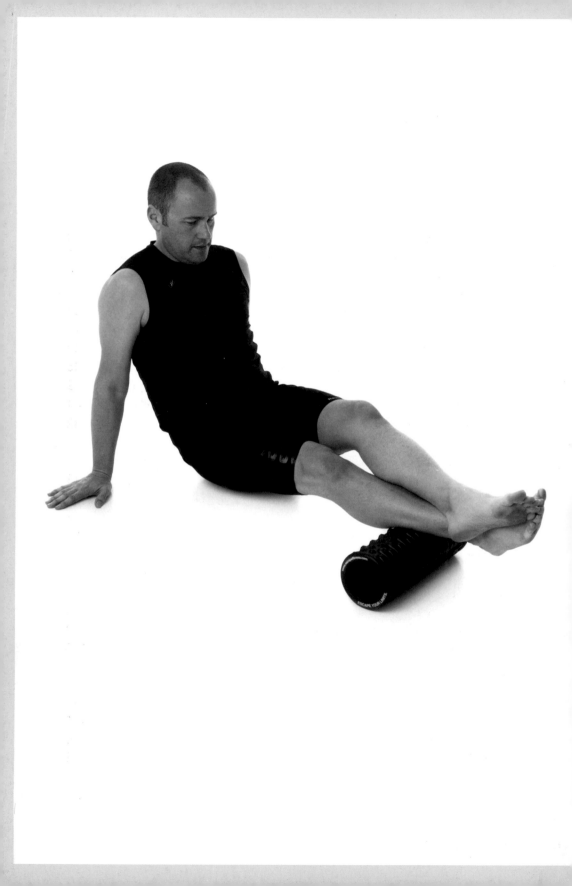

contents

1 the basics of exercising with a foam roller

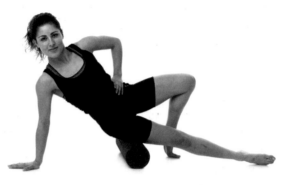

what is foam rolling and how does it work?

Foam rolling is a bit like giving yourself a sports massage. Instead of a masseur's hands applying pressure to relieve muscle tension and discomfort, you apply this yourself. Using your bodyweight on a foam roller you can target problem areas of muscle and fascia (of which more later) and increase your flexibility and recovery time following exercise.

Foam rolling has seen an amazing rise in popularity in the world of health and fitness and has been universally embraced by coaches, professional athletes and those who simply try it and experience almost instant benefits and results. Nothing unusual about that – but foam rolling is different. Most new crazes or trends happen because a product is new, innovative, technical and, more often than not, has a large company behind it spending a fortune on marketing. But with foam rolling the growth in popularity has been 'organic' – via word of mouth rather than due to an advertising campaign. Why is this? Well, foam rolling works. It has a number of benefits, which include pain relief, improved posture, improved performance and, for me the most relevant, manageable, improved and maintainable range of motion in joints. But there isn't a lot of evidence in the fitness industry to tell us why. There are plenty of examples of activities that work but can't be fully explained and even drugs (natural and man-made) that are used globally but aren't fully understood – aspirin being a great example. It's been commercially available since 1899, but even in 1966 it was still unclear how and why it worked, and today there are still discoveries being made into 'new' uses for the drug.

Foam rolling presents us with a similar list of 'unknowns', which are unlikely to be solved any time soon. The reality is that research is generally only done on products by equipment manufacturers who have something to gain (or protect). With foam rolling, few people dispute the feel-good benefits, which in turn means defining the actual physiological process is less urgent than for products that make big claims but struggle to deliver.

So, what are the various theories about how and why foam rolling works? I've put these theories in my personal order of preference.

theory 1: foam rolling softens fascia

Fascia is a fantastic substance that exists throughout the body. Most people understand the function of muscles and some can explain the purpose of ligaments and tendons, but many personal trainers are oblivious to the importance and relevance of fascia throughout the body. Fascia is a fibrous tissue which connects and secures other structures to each other – it's often described as being similar to cling film in that it wraps muscle fibres together. But this description does it a disservice as fascia is far more versatile than this. Here are some of its uses:

- provides a shiny sheath for muscles to slide or glide through during contractions
- suspends organs (especially inter-abdominal objects) inside the torso
- performs a similar function to that of ligaments and tendons to transmit movement from muscles to attachment points on bones.

The theory of how foam rolling affects fascia makes a lot of sense if you first understand that fascia has the ability to adhere (get stuck) to other surfaces but not always in a good way. It has been suggested that fascia itself becomes stiff

9

or 'scarred', which inhibits the ability of the muscles to which it connects to move and function correctly. Similar to how a talented sports masseur can feel changes of texture beneath the skin and target them, foam rolling – often described as a 'poor man's sports massage' – also has a positive effect on fascia.

Now let's talk about ground substance. You may have never heard of this stuff before (I certainly hadn't come across it in all my years as a fitness professional), but it turns out that ground substance is as important as fascia. Fascia is bathed in ground substance, a lubricating fluid/gel that responds positively to movement, pressure and torsion, turning from a thick gel to a fluid. Inactivity makes the ground substance thicken – not a good thing.

The process of foam rolling changes the consistency of ground substance from a thicker gel to a fluid. The medical term for this magical transformation is 'thixotropy'. In my head, ground substance is, therefore, 'the juice that makes you move'! The structure of fascia is a simple mix of collagen, water and lubricating ground substance. If the ground substance hardens due to inactivity, fatigue or postural overload, fluid is forced out of the structure, which results in the closing up of the gaps in the honeycomb formation of the collagen. Foam rolling seems to increase the fluidity of the ground substance, which in turn increases or maintains the fascia's ability to retain fluid in a positive way.

To have this positive effect on fascia with a foam roller, the technique used needs to be made up of: *long, slow, sweeping movements.*

theory 2: foam rolling improves quality of muscle tissue

The idea of 'improving muscle tissue' is a bit vague, I think, and an over-simplification of what happens when we foam roll areas of the body. The theory is similar to the idea of tenderising a piece of meat by hitting it with a hammer, or rolling out dough with a rolling pin. If either of these actually translated to what is happening in the body, we would effectively be suggesting that beating the structure of muscles to pulp is a good thing. But, I think the analogy being used here is the problem – not the process; tenderising dead meat is nothing like massaging muscle.

Muscles create and maintain structural integrity (our posture) by working in conjunction with the muscle opposing it (its antagonist). Without doubt, our posture is the biggest clue that the body gives us about our well-being and the condition of all our soft tissues. Any damage, inflammation or dysfunction will show up 'downstream and upstream' of the actual problem. So, an issue in the foot left untreated will lead to problems in the calf, which can lead to problems around the knee, i.e. upstream. A problem in your lower back may start to manifest itself as an issue in your buttock that then seems to spread down the back of your leg into your hamstring, i.e. downstream. Structural integrity of the muscles produces 'correct' biomechanics, which in effect means that all the muscles, ligaments, tendons and fascia are working as a well-disciplined team rather than as individual heroes.

Foam rolling is basically the self-administered version of 'petrissage', the form of massage where muscles are kneaded deeply and firmly. To generate similar outcomes to 'hands-on' massage, we aren't trying to squash muscles and stretch them out like we do to dough with a rolling pin by constantly changing direction to increase its surface area. Instead, with foam rollers, we should visualise the direction of the muscle between its origin and insertion (the two main attachment points) and roll between those points with as much downward force (pain) as you can cope with. In my experience, foam rolling works best on larger muscles like thighs, hamstrings, calves and the upper back.

To have this positive effect on muscle tissue with a foam roller, the technique used needs to be made up of: *long, slow, sweeping movements following the long axis of the muscle.*

theory 3: foam rolling numbs 'trigger points'

Trigger points (if they actually exist) are 'hot spots' around the body where there is a natural tendency for increased amounts of tension or inflammation where a selection of muscles connect to perform their tasks. Think of these areas as being like a road junction where a number of major roads all cross each other. The roads that carry the most traffic are more likely to become blocked when they are overloaded. You can actually feel this 'congestion' beneath the skin if you apply direct pressure on a trigger point. These hot spots seem to magically reduce in sensitivity when treated with sports massage or foam rolling.

It's argued that there are over 100 potential hot spots around the body (far too many to go into in detail), but if you have a moderate understanding of biomechanics and anatomy, they are easy to identify with your thumb and some careful pressure. You will feel a hard, sensitive nodule. Often a twitch can be felt in the muscle by running your finger perpendicular (at right angles) to the muscle's direction.

Of these 100 hot spots, targeting just six areas with a foam roller should have an overall noticeable effect, not because we are ignoring the other 94 but because these also get attention when rolling the most significant six. From the top, these are:

- pectorals (chest)
- psoas (torso)
- piriformis (buttocks)
- iliotibial (IT) band (outer thigh)
- quadriceps (thighs)
- soleus (lower leg).

These are the muscles most often affected by overuse, fatigue, poor posture and especially sitting down too much, and there are massive benefits to targeting these areas as a whole rather than trying to pinpoint the exact trigger point.

Confusingly, trigger points aren't widely researched or acknowledged by the medical profession as even existing, let alone being responsive to treatment. Many people in the fitness industry would be surprised by this as the term 'trigger point' is commonly used, but this is another case of a method being widely prescribed without personal trainers questioning the source. However, while there is much scepticism, I can honestly say, from personal experience and having witnessed improvements with clients, I know that targeting these spots is a worthwhile exercise. In the portfolio of moves I have included some 'micro-isolation' moves that pinpoint these hot spots, in addition to the rolling techniques that address wider areas of muscle fibres.

To have this positive effect on trigger points with a foam roller, the technique used needs to be made up of: *small repetitive movements on the trigger points ('hot spots') around the body.*

theory 4: foam rolling breaks up scar tissue

Scar tissue sounds really dramatic but tissue can be scarred quite easily, to varying degrees. At the worst end of the spectrum are muscles that have been ruptured (completely torn apart) and will have visible and feelable permanent scar tissue. While massage and foam rolling will seem to improve its functionality, scar tissue is also purposefully less malleable than the original fibres as a means of protecting that area from repeat tearing. The downside of this protective reaction by the body is that the pathway of nerves can become blocked, leading to referred pain symptoms, i.e. pain either upstream or downstream from the problem. At the other end of the spectrum, muscle fibres are damaged and scar on a regular basis if you perform intense physical activity. The most common example of this is DOMS (delayed onset muscle soreness). We used to think that DOMS was trapped lactic acid but that theory has been dismissed, and it is now thought to be due to tiny tears in the muscle. Sports massage has for many years proved an effective solution to managing this type of damage. If we treat foam rolling as in essence a self-administered sports massage, it follows that the benefits will be similar. Realistically, however, scar tissue won't disappear completely (if it did, surgeons around the world would be recommending massage to improve their results after surgery). Scar tissue is a mass of fibres that are more randomly connected than their unscarred predecessors. Healthy fibres are more uniform, fitting together neatly next to each other and moving freely against each other, with all of their cells having a good blood supply. Scar tissue in comparison is less 'organised', is matted together and has a poorer blood supply.

A foam roller is a very blunt weapon so it's hard to roll on very specific spots. This means, unless you have a large area of scar tissue that is all parallel to the surface of the skin, it's unlikely you will be able to pinpoint the spot with a roller. This is why also having a hard ball like a lacrosse or cricket ball to roll on is good because you can get very specific with the spot that you want to target. However, scar tissue will always be scar tissue no matter how much attention you give it, so, logically, I am more inclined to think that working on the entire muscle around a scarred area is more productive than just beating up the damaged spot.

To have this positive effect on scar tissue with a foam roller, the technique used needs to be made up of: *long, slow, sweeping movements following the long axis of the muscle with shorter sweeps across and 'against the grain' of the muscle fibres.*

theory 5: foam rolling affects the way the central nervous system deals with pain with the release of chemicals from the brain

This is the newest theory associated with using foam rollers and it is radically different from all the others. Brace yourself, this starts out sounding technical!

Diffuse noxious inhibitory control (DNIC) is one of several varieties of chemical reactions, by which the brain adjusts the 'volume' of pain/danger signals that originate in the body. DNIC means that the brain blocks pain signals from travelling up the spinal cord to the brain once it has detected that there is something causing pain downstream. DNIC is triggered by a sustained sensation, such as immersing your hand in cold water, suppressing the pain not just from the cold wet area, but in distant areas as well. In other words, if your foot hurts, and you put your hand in iced water until it numbs, the resulting DNIC will cause both the hand and the foot to hurt less. The effect is temporary, of course, which is why I'm not convinced that DNIC is the only theory behind the positive results of foam rolling. For example, when I roll I feel better throughout the entire day whereas, taking the cold water analogy, the pain relief from DNIC is only as temporary as the coldness. I'm absolutely not dismissing it, as the reality is there has been more research done on pain management than there will ever be into the effects of rolling.

To my knowledge no proper research has yet been done to test chemical reactions whilst foam rolling, so until a large scale study* is completed specifically to explore this I think it's best to acknowledge DNIC but put more faith in the theory that foam rolling creates mechanical outcomes rather than chemical peaks and troughs.

To clarify, the theory behind DNIC is that, if there is pain downstream, the brain will send a response down the spinal cord to deal with it. For example, if you roll your buttocks and it hurts (a nice hurt, but still it hurts), that info is sent to the brain suggesting there is pain/danger in that particular area. In response the brain, knowing that it is a 'good pain', sends chemicals down the spinal cord to convince the body part that actually all is well, allowing you to continue.

To have this positive effect on a muscle with a foam roller, the technique used needs to be: *on large areas. Theoretically, all foam rolling will induce this response as long as 'pain' is inflicted on areas of the body, so, logically, the bigger the area the better as it will induce a greater response from the brain.*

You may have heard the phrase self-myofascial release (SMR) used when foam rolling is discussed. For clarity SMR is the general term used to describe most types of manual therapy that is looking to have an effect upon the soft tissue under the skin, e.g. massage with hands, rollers or electronic devices – so for clarity all foam rolling activities are SMR but not all SMR is foam rolling.

* Specific studies would require rolling to be performed whilst the participant was hooked up to a monitoring device such as an MRI scanner.

the S.A.F.E. trainer system
(Simple, Achievable, Functional Exercise)

We need to exercise our bodies in a way that is achievable, effective and, most of all, sustainable so that the method becomes part of our lifestyle, rather than an inconvenience.

In a perfect world everyone would be able to lift their own bodyweight above their head, have ideal body fat levels and be able to run a four-minute mile. Any one of these goals is achievable if you are highly motivated and have very few other commitments in your life, but the reality is that most people are so far off this state of perfection that the biggest challenge is either starting an exercise programme or staying committed and engaged with a method of training for long enough to see any kind of improvement.

Exercise is in many ways a perfect product, because it has very few negative side effects, it is cheap to do and highly versatile. But so many high-profile, quick-fix programmes and products make exercise sound easy, as though it is a magic wand that once waved will bring near instant results. And with the fitness industry constantly driven by innovation in products and methods, the diverse and sometimes bewildering amount of advice available makes it all too easy to be overwhelmed, and, if you are not careful in choosing your methods, all too easy to cause yourself harm. The truth is that many training programmes and methods will theoretically work, but the level of commitment needed is so high that when you add in work and family responsibilities, stress and other demands upon time, most of us simply cannot stick to a plan.

I also find that those programmes which seem too good to be true usually have a series of components that are not explicit in the headline, but are required to achieve the spectacular results it boasts about. So you sign up to a workout programme claiming: 'Instant fat loss – ultra 60 second workout!' only to find that to achieve the promised weight loss you have to go on an impossible 500-calorie-a-day diet. These methods also assume that everybody is fairly perfect already; by this I mean they don't have any injuries, they are strong, mobile and flexible and have a cardiovascular system that will soak up anaerobic training from day one. If these people are out there, I don't see them walking up and down the average high street. There is a real need to approach fitness in a more down-to-earth, less sensationalist way. We need to exercise our bodies in a manner that is achievable, effective and, most of all, sustainable so that the method becomes part of our lifestyle, rather than an inconvenience.

My S.A.F.E. trainer system (Simple, Achievable, Functional Exercise) is all of these things. It is based on 25+ years of personal training experience, including many thousands of hours of coaching, lifting, running, jumping and stretching with people from all walks of life, from the average man or woman to elite athletes. My system respects the natural way that the body adapts to activity and creates a perfect physiological learning curve.

The S.A.F.E. trainer approach mimics components of human performance. I am sure that you will recognise the saying 'You have to walk before you can run'. This is the epitome of my approach, because when a client says they want to run or jump, the first thing I have to establish as a personal trainer is that they are at least already at the walking stage. This means that everything I can influence is working well enough to be challenged in training sessions. Foam rolling has been a revelation in this whole process as over the years I have met so many people who have just put up with aches and pains and accepted them as being the norm, and so are rather miffed when you tell them that they really aren't as fit or able to train in the way they think they should be. However, by highlighting their 'hot spots' and putting them through rather painful foam rolling sessions, they usually get the message that loading (with weights) and fatiguing already 'damaged' fibres will only be counterproductive.

As I have worked with many of my clients now for over two decades, clearly they find my approach productive and a worthwhile investment. With this in mind, my aim is to condense 25 years' experience of training my own body and, more importantly, 25 years' experience as a personal trainer and many thousands of hours of training the bodies of other people into this book. With the luxury of being able to reflect on my experiences as a 'proper' qualified teacher who has trained many hundreds, perhaps thousands, of other personal trainers, all this means that my methodology is pretty much tried and tested. Yes, I have trained A-list celebrities (which seems to be a goal for many personal trainers), but in reality it's like any other 'day in the office'. I've also trained royalty and plenty of international sports superstars, but, to me, every training session boils down to a similar experience for both me and my client: they want to get maximum results from the time they are prepared to invest in exercise, and I want to make sure that I exceed their expectations and give them a return on their investment. Every exercise I select for their session, therefore, has to have earned its place in the programme, and every teaching point that I provide needs to be worthwhile and have a positive outcome. I also don't go in for 'beastings' or 'destroying' people. The reality is, apart from those few who actually earn their living from their body, most people have to be able to function and go about their everyday business the day after each session. Even though I know many PTs revel in the fact that they 'smash' their client, I tend to think that exercise only really has an effect if it becomes a habit. In essence, my teaching style could almost be described as persuasive and also minimalist. While I certainly wouldn't let you get away with doing things wrong, I have the rational that to make health and fitness a long-term part of your life means accepting that not hitting perfection every time is better than not bothering in the first place – which is why 'if you're moving, you're improving' tends to be my tagline. As I bound into my third decade in the fitness industry I know that knowledge is subjective and that the availability of information hasn't made any difference to the population's fitness levels as a whole, so I don't go in for trying to show you how clever I am when all that is required are clear, concise constructive instructions to get the job done.

I learned this lesson many years ago when I was hired as personal trainer to a professor of medicine. She is uber-intelligent with a complete disinterest in trivia and I became resigned to the fact there was absolutely nothing I could say about the function of the body or the effects of exercise that she didn't already know – gulp! But what I could do was assess her current level of ability and take her on the shortest, safest and most effective route to an improved level of fitness. Twenty years on having run, rode, swam, rollerbladed and hiked together, and now of course foam rolled together, I am still keeping her engaged in the pursuit and benefits of exercise by finding new ways to help her enjoy the time we spend training together (and she lets me drive her Aston Martin DB5, which is an added bonus)!

So, where does foam rolling fit in? Well, with the other 'Total Workout' books in the series, the exercises progress in difficulty, intensity and complexity through three stages, which are: firstly 'stability', progressing to 'strength' then peaking with 'power'. These three stages have a direct correlation with activity that you do in everyday life and many sports. But foam rolling is about enhancing our ability to do these activities, rather than replicating them in the session by challenging the body progressively to respond and improve. Our aim with the foam roller is to recondition (or restore) the soft tissues of the body (muscle, fascia and ground matter) to function at their best. I still like to see logical progressions, but it's more for user tolerance levels (foam rolling can feel painful when you start) rather than ability. In effect, I'm talking about progressions relating to 'needs' of the tissue rather than 'wants' of a participant. I'll talk about the actual terminology later but as a preview everything we do in the early stage is about 'erasing pain', then once you have established a decent level of tolerance to foam rolling we 'invest (time to mobilise)', and ultimately continue the process forever as we 'maintain'.

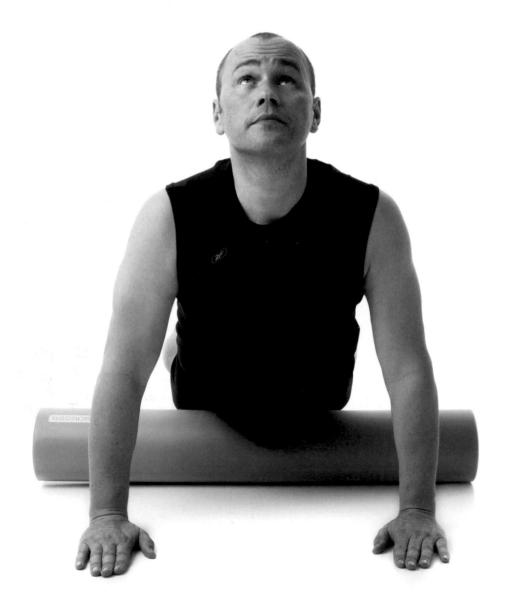

how to use this book

Committing time to using a foam roller properly should be considered as an investment in your well-being. Clearly, the amount of time you spend doing it will dictate the outcomes, however, I think that with all pieces of fitness equipment there can be a novelty factor (maybe it looks cool or is innovative), which makes you want to use it. But with a foam roller it's difficult to get excited about what is, in most cases, just a clever chunk of foam. Add to this the fact that when you start rolling your neglected or fatigued muscles it will probably be painful – and potentially any novelty of foam rolling could wear off pretty quickly. My approach is this: I really want you to try and build foam rolling into your daily routine rather than have it 'take over' for a short period of time only to be forgotten about in a few weeks.

Imagine that instead of cleaning your teeth every day you stopped and only gave them a really good cleaning session once a week. By the second day, you would start to notice the grime; by the third and fourth, things would be starting to feel pretty rough; and by the seventh day, they would be crying out for attention. Our soft tissue is going to respond in exactly the same way except, instead of having rough teeth and bad breath, you won't notice the tissue fatigue caused by prolonged exercise creeping up on you.

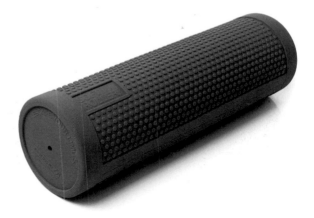

FAQs

These are the most common questions that fitness trainers are asked in relation to exercising with a foam roller.

What type and size roller do I need? Long, short, hard, soft, hollow or lumpy?

High density foam

These are the original style of foam roller that have been available since the 1980s, and whilst all products in this category of equipment are described as being 'foam' rollers these days it's only the high density foam versions that are made of a substance most people would consider to be actual foam. It has visible air holes in it, which make it capable of deforming under pressure then regaining its original shape when released in the same way that a foam mattress does. High-density foam is made from an oil-based product and has tiny air holes in it. All rollers of this type are the softest and therefore the least painful, making them ideal for beginners and maintenance work. I like the longer versions as they are particularly good for working the upper back area, but the short versions can be used for all the exercises in this book. Some of these rollers are cheaper than others but be aware that the cheapest ones, open cell foam, lose their shape quicker than the slightly more expensive closed cell foam, they also don't absorb sweat, which has got to be a good enough reason to spend that little extra.

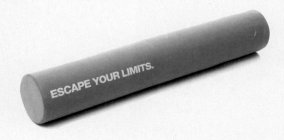

EVA (ethylene vinyl acetate)

This is the type of roller you are most likely to find in a commercial gym because they last for ages without losing their shape or firmness. Most people describe the material of the roller as rubber or vinyl rather than foam, but technically because it's made by trapping gas within the EVA during manufacturing, it is classed as foam. They are invariably harder than the high-density foam version, but only slightly. Also, because of the characteristics of the material, they can be made in a variety of diameters, but I find 12–15cm the most versatile.

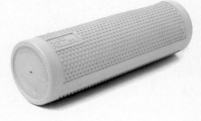

Rumble roller

If foam rolling was a competitive sport, this would be the most extreme version. This is a solid pipe roller with an outer coating of extremely prominent peaks (I'd say spikes but they don't have points on). These peaks can be used to target small hot spots. Because your bodyweight is in contact with a smaller surface area (just the peaks) when you roll large areas of the body, it hurts more than with any other type of roller – only for the brave and experienced.

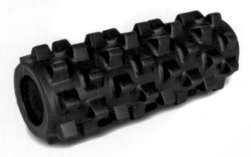

Pipe roller/ridge roller

This is the one I use most. It is a solid pipe covered in a layer of EVA foam. This dual component product is considered by those in the know to be the gold standard of roller as it seems to deliver the right amount of pain (neural feedback), but also the EVA foam coating seems more bearable for beginners as well as advanced (conditioned) users. This is the roller featured in some of our photographs. The 'ridge roller' is thus named as it has a combination of ridges and grooves across its surface, which you can feel in a nice way, rather than increasing the pain. In fact, the thinking is that the ridges mimic the fingertips of a masseur, making this truly the poor man's sports massage. Again the longer versions are best for doing the upper back but the short ones are better for total body work as you can get into tighter spots with them (for example, the inner thigh).

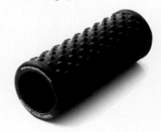

Balls

Not actually a roller but equally as useful for rolling on. Some of the exercises done on a roller take on a completely different level of intensity when performed on a ball. You can buy balls designed for therapy but most users will get good results using a solid ball like a lacrosse ball (which is slightly larger than a cricket ball). Some people go a stage further by taping two balls together to create something that looks like a very large unshelled peanut. This can be used for rolling straight down the spine (one ball either side of the vertebrae). Personally I find these extremely intense and feel they get too close to bones in my spine so I use a slightly more expensive option made out of EVA foam.

How often should I be rolling?

Ideally, roll every day, I say. This might sound onerous but once you have practised and established the areas of the body, which seem to require constant attention you will only be doing 15 minutes per session. There's no need to get changed in to workout gear or even get dressed if you are doing it at home! Realistically I know that most people want to negotiate down from optimal to minimal, but I'm not going to give a token number like three times per week for 15 mins as this defeats the object of foam rolling. With rolling, you will get out exactly as much as you put in – so you decide.

It really hurts, should I stop?

It will hurt, but actually, if you tell yourself that it is doing you good, it becomes a 'nice pain'. If the pain is unbearable then clearly you should stop. However, if

I was next to you, I would most likely try to encourage you to stick with it and do at least 5–6 slow rolls on the hot spot before giving up as the pain generally diminishes after the first couple of repetitions.

Will I get bruises from rolling?
In my experience, no. Some people get some redness where they have been applying pressure but this is temporary.

Is foam rolling an alternative to regular stretching?
Yes, if by regular stretching you mean static stretches rather than dynamic stretching. Static stretches are a favourite of people who are already flexible. However, there is now increasing debate as to the benefits of developing elongated muscles rather than allowing them to maintain mechanical tension to keep the skeleton upright. Basically, if you do static stretches in moderation, you will maintain mechanical tension, but if you choose to constantly stretch your favourite muscle (for example, the hamstring), then this will become saggy compared to its opposite muscle (the quadriceps). I don't want to oversimplify the explanation but think of it like this: if you have a woollen sweater and keep pulling at just one sleeve, then that sleeve will become distorted compared to the other one. So, unless you are extremely methodical and stretch everywhere consistently, you will end up out of balance. However, due to the 'mechanical' effect of foam rolling, I don't think the same can be said about it.

Which direction should I roll?
Most of the time we roll along the longest axis of the muscle. So, for example, with the quadriceps, we go from knee to hip and back again. However, muscle and certainly not fascia don't conform to being positioned in neat symmetrical patterns so using the anatomical centre line* of the body as a reference point we roll parallel, 30, 45 and 90 degrees to it. If we were massaging with hands rather than with a roller, we would apply more pressure when going towards the heart and less on the return stroke; however, with rolling it is virtually impossible to be this subtle so we keep the pressure constant.

How fast should I move?
Start slow and then as you improve get slower! Seriously, you must try and create a mind-body connection when rolling. If you just want to get it over with, you

*the anatomical centre line cuts the body in half from the nose to the centre of the groin.

will invariably just be going through the motions, which is about as much use as having a jar of vitamins in your cupboard but never taking them. As a guide, when rolling the front of your thighs each motion should take approximately 3 seconds – that might not sound long but there are guys who can run 30 metres in that amount of time, so count it in your head as you roll and I expect you will be going much slower than when you don't apply some discipline.

What are trigger points?

As touched upon earlier (see page 11), trigger points are hot spots spread around the body where there is a natural tendency for increased amounts of tension or inflammation, generally where a selection of muscles attach via a tendon to perform their tasks; they also correspond with many of the known acupressure points. Conservatively there are over 100 potential trigger points around the body and, even if you have no understanding of biomechanics and anatomy, they are easy to identify with your thumb/finger and some pressure. The easiest to find on yourself is where the pectoral major muscle connects to the shoulder: put your finger on your collar bone near your shoulder then move down and slightly back towards the body's centre line where it feels soft then press firmly – ouch! That's a trigger point, you may even feel the sensation go all the way down your arm to your hand.

What's the one trade secret that we should all adhere to?

Be aware of your hydration levels. We are trying to manage/reduce inflammation and enhance tissue function, both of which are reliant on optimal hydration levels. So ensure that you are never thirsty when you are foam rolling – ideally drink little and often and get to know your own needs.

finding your starting point

Before starting any exercise programme, test your body against the fitness checklist: mobility, flexibility, muscle recruitment and strength.

If any of these vital components are neglected, it will have a knock-on effect on your progress. For example, while you may have the raw strength in your quadriceps to squat with a heavy weight, if you do not have a full range of motion in the ankle joints and sufficient flexibility in the calf muscles, then your squat will inevitably be of poor quality. Likewise, in gyms it is common to see men who have overtrained their chest muscles to such an extent that they can no longer achieve scapular retraction (they are round shouldered and therefore demonstrate poor technique in moves that require them to raise their arms above their heads). I realise I mention strength training a number of times in this section and this type of exercise might not be on your agenda, and that's fine. I mention it because foam rolling is something that some readers will be doing to resolve issues they have due to not doing any structured exercise whilst others will be integrating rolling into an existing regime and to help improve their performance either in the gym or in another performance environment. Basically the beauty of using the foam rolling techniques I describe later is that they complement everything and conflict with nothing.

This type of checklist is traditionally the most overlooked component of health screening and, while testing weight, body-fat levels and cardiac performance is now a regular occurrence in the fitness industry, the introduction of screening for quality of movement has taken a much longer time to become a priority. This, can be as simple as looking in the mirror.

There is no better summary of how important our ability to move freely is than in one of my favourite sayings: 'Use it or lose it'. This says it all – if you don't use the body to perform physical tasks it will more likely deteriorate rather than just stay the same.

It may be no coincidence that assessing movement quality has grown in importance today for athletes and fitness enthusiasts at the same pace as the popularity of functional training – rightly so because if you don't assess yourself then how can you know what areas of functionality you need to work on most? Before functional training became a key component of progressive fitness programmes all the progressions related to increasing duration and intensity and resistance, however now the quality of movement has become of equal importance.

Today, the assessment of 'functional movement', or biomechanical screening, is its own specialised industry within the world of fitness. Those working in ortho-paedics and conventional medical rehabilitation have always followed some form of standardised assessment where they test the function of the nerves, muscles and bones before forming an opinion of a patient's condition. Becoming a trained practitioner takes many years of study and practice. Not only must a practitioner gain knowledge of a wide spectrum of potential conditions, but just as importantly they must understand when and how to treat their patient, or when they need to refer them to other colleagues in the medical profession.

Having been subjected to and taught many different approaches to movement screening, in my mind, the challenge isn't establishing there is something 'wrong', rather it is knowing what to do to rectify the issue.

assess, don't guess

Of all the different types of exercise I use with clients the one element that they always comment on most positively is the functional movement screening.

As a personal trainer I am used to being given a wish list by new clients, which if I'm honest usually contains similar requests from person to person: lose weight, get stronger, improve muscle definition, etc. are all common goals, but never have I had someone actually ask for their quality of movement to be improved – why is this? I think it must be because first they don't realise they are walking around with so many stored up 'issues' and that ignoring them is likely to cause problems in the future. It's like thinking that you can build a house by putting the roof up first without building the walls or sorting out the foundations. So, whilst it's not on most people's shopping list, assessing movement quality is probably the one way I am able to prove the benefits of my training methods either in the first few weeks or months of working with a client. If you don't assess then you are just guessing.

I first started including a functional movement screen assessment for new clients in the 1990s, and it quickly became an essential component of getting to know clients better and also enabled me to monitor improvements. Also, being a lot younger back then, and in almost permanent hard training mode I hadn't realised until I started doing assessments that my own body was riddled with painful triggers and prone to imbalances that would be having an effect upon my performance, so surely so would my clients. Jump forwards 30 years and foam rolling has helped refine this process because whilst the two tests described in this section (standing twist test and the overhead squat test) give you visual feedback about whether everything is moving and working well, using a foam roller enhances the critique process enormously as now it is possible to feel issues under the skin as well as seeing them interrupting movement patterns.

mobility and flexibility

The most common problem limiting quality of movement in the average person is a lack of mobility and flexibility, which can be provisionally tested using the standing twist and the overhead squat assessment (see pages 29–30).

To understand why mobility is key to human movement, think how as babies we start to move independently. We are born with mobility and flexibility, then we progressively develop stability, balance and then increasing amounts of strength.

The following two mobility tests challenge the entire length of the kinetic chain (actions and reaction to force that occur throughout the bones, muscles and nerves whenever dynamic motion or force is required from the body). They also help to reveal if you are ready to move beyond bodyweight-derived exercises and begin adding the additional loads inflicted upon the body by equipment such as kettlebells, dumbbells and barbells but also strength machines and anything that requires you to exert a force for example running or riding up steep hills. This test focuses on the following key areas of the shoulders: the mid-thoracic spine, pelvis, knees, ankles and feet. Any limitation of mobility, flexibility or strength in these areas will show up as either an inability to move smoothly through the exercise or an inability to hold the body in the desired position.

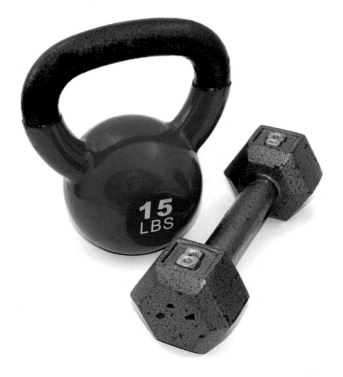

Test 1 standing twist

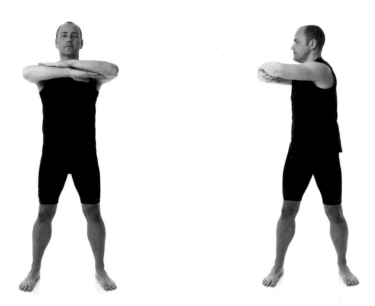

This is the less dramatic of the two mobility tests and serves to highlight whether you have any pain that only presents when you move through the outer regions of your range of movement, and also if you have a similar range of motion between rotations on the left and right sides of your body.

- Stand with your feet beneath your hips.
- Raise your arms to chest height then rotate as far as you can to the right, noting how far you can twist.
- Repeat the movement to the left.
- Perform the movement slowly so that no 'extra twist' is achieved using speed and momentum.

Your observation is trying to identify any pain and/or restriction of movement. If you find either, it might be the case that this reduces after a warm-up or a few additional repetitions of this particular movement. If you continue to experience pain, you should consider having it assessed by a physiotherapist or sports therapist.

Test 2 Overhead squat (OHS)

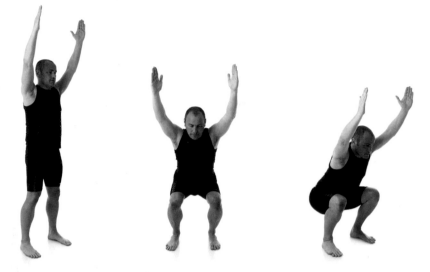

I've used the OHS test over 5000 times as part of my S.A.F.E. approach to exercise and have found it to be the quickest and easiest way of looking at basic joint and muscle function without getting drawn into speculative diagnosis of what is and isn't working properly. If you can perform this move without any pain or restriction, then you will find most of the moves in this book achievable. There is no pass or fail, rather you will fall into one of two categories: 'good' or 'could do better'. If you cannot achieve any of the key requirements of the OHS move, then it is your body's way of flagging up that you are tight and/or weak in that particular area. This in turn could mean you have an imbalance, pain or an untreated injury, which may not prevent you from exercising, but you should probably get checked out by a physiotherapist or sports therapist.

Perform this exercise barefoot and in front of a full-length mirror so that you can gain maximum information from the observation of your whole body. Also refer to Table 1 for a list of key body regions to observe during the test. (This move also doubles up as a brilliant warm-up for many types of exercise including lifting weights.)

- Stand with feet pointing straight ahead and at hip width.
- Have your hands in the 'thumbs-up position' and raise your arms above your head, keeping them straight, into the top of a 'Y' position (with your body being the bottom of the 'Y'). Your arms are in the correct position when they are back far enough to disappear from your peripheral vision.

- The squat down is slow and deep, so take a slow count of six to get down by bending your knees. The reason we go slowly is so you do not allow gravity to take over and merely slump down. You also get a chance to see and feel how everything is moving through the six key areas.

The magic of this move is that you will be able to see and feel where your problem spots are and, even better, the test becomes the solution, as simply performing it regularly helps with your quality of movement. Stretch out any area that feels tight and aim to work any area that feels weak.

Table 1 Key body regions to observe in the overhead squat

Body region	Good position	Bad position
Neck		
Shoulders		
Mid-thoracic spine		
Hips		

Knees		
Ankles and feet		

As you perform the OHS you are looking for control and symmetry throughout and certain key indicators that all is well:

- **Neck:** You keep good control over your head movements and are able to maintain the arm lift without pain in the neck.
- **Shoulders:** In the start position and throughout the move you are aiming to have both arms lifted above the head and retracted enough so that they are outside your peripheral vision (especially when you are in the deep part of the squat). In addition to observing the shoulders look up at your arms to the hands – throughout the OHS you should aim to have your thumbs pointing behind you.
- **Mid-thoracic spine:** There is no instruction to keep your back straight, so in this area of the body you are looking for 'flow' rather than clunking movements.
- **Hips:** Imagine a straight line drawn directly down the centre of your body. Around the hips you are looking to see if you shift your weight habitually to one side, rather than keeping it evenly spread between both sides.
- **Knees:** The most common observation is the knees touching during the OHS, suggesting a weakness in the glutes. Less common is the knees parting, showing weakness in the inner thigh. Good technique is when your knees move forwards as you bend the legs. Note that clicking and crunching noises don't always suggest a problem unless they are accompanied by pain.
- **Ankles and feet:** The most obvious issue is the heels lifting from the floor, suggesting short Achilles and calf muscles. Less obvious are the flattening of the foot arches that cause the feet to roll inward (overpronation) or the foot rolling outward (underpronation). Ideally, the foot should be in a neutral position.

If when you do the OHS in front of the mirror you observe any of these signals with your kinetic chain (the actions and reaction to force that occur throughout the bones, muscles and nerves whenever dynamic motion or force is required from the body), it really isn't the end of the world, in fact, most people find that they are tight in some areas (if not all of them) when they first try this test. The absolutely fantastic news is that if you do spot any issues, performing the OHS as an exercise, rather than merely a test, will improve your movement pattern, joint range and muscle actions over time.

overhead squat: the results

My rule is that if you can perform a perfect OHS, with none of the key warning signs listed above, then you are ready to embark on virtually any type of training programme using a variety of equipment or challenges, and incorporating foam rolling into this regime will enhance the entire process. In this incidence foam rolling will conflict with nothing else that you do and complement everything.

However if you don't achieve a perfect score then think about the OHS as flagging up weaknesses when you are only moving your bodyweight so adding weight or pressure is most likely to compound the poor movement quality that you have developed. Fix the problem then you can rest assured that you aren't putting force through joints that are already stressed. So, use the OHS as a guide to whether your body is as ready as your mind is.

If you find by doing the OHS that your body is not ready for some types of sports or intense activities, rest assured, it is ready for foam rolling. Remember foam rolling complements everything and conflicts with nothing.

fascia – the unsung hero

So what is the big deal with fascia? Fascia is a whitish pink fibrous tissue in appearance, which can range from being so thin that it is transparent to being so thick that it looks like a thick gristly tendon. Found throughout the body, it is a fantastic substance which connects and secures other structures to each other, but if it becomes stiff or scarred, it can inhibit the ability of the connecting muscles to move and function correctly.

A good sports masseur can feel changes of texture beneath the skin, which have a correlation with heightened levels of pain for the patient when touched using light or firm targeted pressure. These sensitive areas can either be due to inflammation or adhesions (internal scar tissue); the worst adhesions can even adhere themselves to the inside of our skin, making it feel oddly connected to the surface beneath it. Recreating this hands-on action with a foam roller can therefore also have instant results. As such, whilst the location of muscles give us

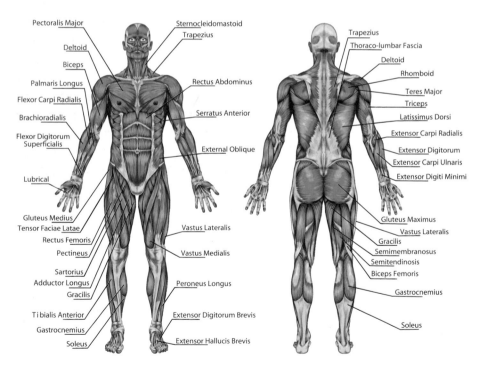

Figure 1 Muscles and fascia

the best method for 'mapping' the body, the presence and position of fascia was a big consideration when I developed the techniques in the portfolio of moves.

The drawing in Figure 1 illustrates in red the way that muscles are positioned and connect on to the human skeleton, the white sections depict areas that are dominated either by thick fascia or ligament/tendons. However, the illustration doesn't quite do justice to the amount of fascia that covers our muscle beneath the skin. So why have we not highlighted the fascia when clearly it is of such importance? Beneath our skin in some form or another, fascia is everywhere, either covering the largest expanses of skeletal muscle or by being secreted in between the grooves formed where one muscle passes close to another – so to illustrate the fascia we would have to wrap the entire body with a white film, but of course by doing that we would be obscuring the muscles so where you see red or white on the drawing please assume there is also a presence of fascia.

Ground substance (rarely even heard mentioned among experienced PTs) is another consideration as to why 'working on' fascia is one of my goals. Once you know about ground substance (see page 10), foam rolling makes absolute sense. As mentioned before, the structure of fascia is simply a mix of collagen, water and lubricating ground substance. If the ground substance hardens due to inactivity, fatigue or postural overload, fluid is forced out of the structure, which results in gaps closing up in the honeycomb formation of the collagen. Foam rolling, it seems, increases the fluidity of the ground substance, which in turn increases or maintains the fascia's ability to retain fluid in a positive way. This is why I specifically mention hydration levels in the FAQ section: if you don't have the right amount of fluid in you, you can't expect fluid-dependent components of the body to function well. Neglect or ignore fascia and it will turn into an invisible villain in your body, making you feel at best average. Engorge it with water and massage it often and it will do you its greatest service by simply getting on with its job.

foam rolling to wipe away pain and unlock performance

Foam rolling could be the magic wand that improves your functional strength. All movements that we do in training or everyday life can be classified as either isolation or integration moves. The vast majority of isolation moves have been created/invented to work specific muscles on their own, with the primary intention of fatiguing that muscle by working it in isolation, usually moving only one joint of the skeleton. Integration, or compound moves are less of an invention and more of an adaptation of movement patterns that we perform in everyday life. They are designed to work groups of muscles across multiple joints all at the same time.

In real life we never isolate – therefore mobility of joints, flexibility of muscles and the fascia play a key role in every movement that we make. Even when only a few joints are moving there is a massive number of muscles bracing throughout the body to let the prime muscles do their job, and part of that bracing is facilitated by fascia. Everything, and I mean everything, we do boils down to the following key movements:

- push
- pull
- twist
- squat
- lunge
- bend
- walk
- run
- jump.

Despite the OHS being a relatively passive movement all the muscles it tests have a direct correlation to your ability to function well when doing any of the nine key human movements. To push effectively you must have stability in the low, mid and upper spine. To pull either your own bodyweight or an external load it becomes irrelevant how strong your limbs are if you cannot simultaneously activate muscles in the torso to stabilise the spine. Being able to stabilise all these areas of the spine is tested by the OHS. To twist and bend you need to be able to stabilise firstly from the spine and then downstream into the hips and

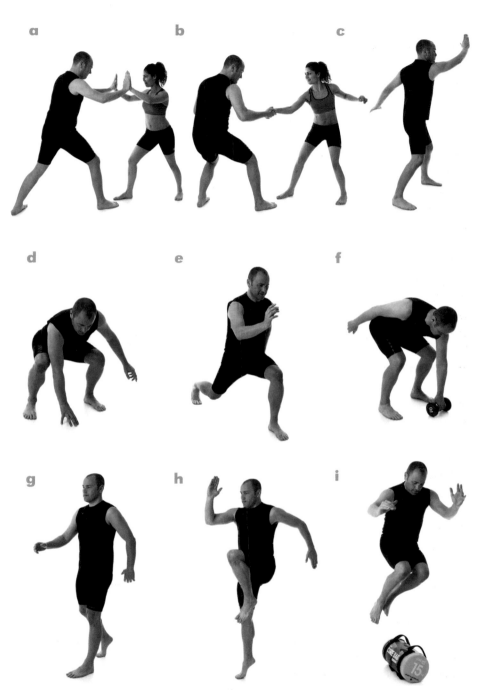

Figure 2 The nine basic human movement patterns: (a) push, (b) pull, (c) twist, (d) squat, (e) lunge, (f) bend, (g) walk, (h) run and (i) jump

pelvis. Most importantly to squat, lunge, walk, run and jump you can have strong muscles in you lower body but if you don't have the ability to stabilise (which is what we are testing with the OHS) then this strength becomes unmanageable.

When I walk down the street behind people, it amazes me how many people have limps, hunched shoulders and a whole host of imbalances and other oddities as part of their regular walking action. Assuming these irregular gaits aren't caused by some type of attitude or self-imposed swagger then the most likely reason is that these people are living with pain and have adapted their gait to minimise any pain radiating from soft tissue (or, of course, arthritic bones – something that won't benefit from rolling).

Pain will always cause a reaction from your body, but it doesn't always have to be an instant traumatic injury that provokes the reaction. Pain from soft tissue injuries can creep up gradually so that a sufferer gradually adapts the way they move to help tolerate the pain. I use the overhead squat (OHS, see page 30) to assess quality of movement in my clients and it took hundreds of OHS assessments before I was able to instinctively look at how a person moved or to 'read' how their movement patterns related to aches, pains and restrictions, so do not worry if you struggle to understand what you are looking for at first. But if you use the OHS as guidance rather than treating it as a diagnosis, then you have the right approach. Remember that the OHS assessment is fantastic because everything we do boils down to the nine key movements. The OHS is not just a test but also part of the cure: if you aim to perform the best quality of movement that you can when doing it, together with the introduction of regular foam rolling you really will be waving a magic wand over your aches and pains.

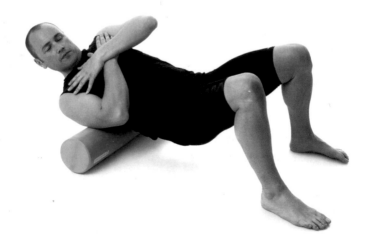

first you need to find your hot spots and erase pain from them with micro rolls

The first time you 'roll' you will undoubtedly think that you are doing something wrong as it is often very painful. For most people the most sensitive areas of your body are best described as 'hot spots' (or trigger points). As we've discussed already, these hot spots are spread throughout the body where there is a natural tendency for higher amounts of tension or inflammation – generally they are where a selection of muscles or tendons attach to or cross multiple joints. A good way to visualise hot spots is to think of them like a junction where multiple busy roads meet – invariably there will be congestion in that area, due to the volume of traffic. This translates to these spots being amongst the most painful (but productive) areas to foam roll. So for the 'find it' phase, concentrate on these sensitive areas until you feel that you have 'erased the pain'. This period can and should be viewed as a process of damage limitation, because if you hadn't decided that foam rolling was something you wanted to add to your body maintenance regime, you would have gradually been storing up trouble for the future.

Now, of course everybody is different but the following areas will be most likely where you find your 'hottest' hot spots and where you will need immediate attention. From the ground up they are:

- gastrocnemius (calf)
- IT band (runs down the side of the outer thigh)
- piriformis (found in the lower buttock)
- quadriceps/hip flexors (thighs and hips)
- erector spinae (runs down the back of the spine)
- pectoralis (chest).

These are the first exercises shown in the portfolio of moves (beginning on page 47). Each of these small areas need to be pinpointed and slowly rolled for 1–2 minutes each ... yes, 1–2 minutes each! Any shorter period at this stage of your training will have significantly less benefit – foam rolling shouldn't be compared to static stretching as holding a static stretch for two minutes has no greater benefit than holding it for one. Foam rolling is entirely different because it's dynamic and, whilst I don't actually count them, we are performing repetitions.

I refer to these exercises as 'micro rolls' because you are targeting only very small spots of discomfort rather than rolling entire sections of the body – those come later and I call them macro rolls because they condition large areas of the body with each passing over the roller. The speed that you perform each roll is also important. It needs to be slow but not hesitant: for example, to roll the gastrocnemius at the appropriate speed would take four seconds (that's two seconds in each direction), whilst to roll a longer section of the body, such as the erector spinae, needs more like six seconds (three up, three down). Don't worry – timings are noted next to each of the moves in the portfolio.

How often should you perform the moves from this section? The best answer is as often as you can – I have seen other trainers advise that you roll 3–5 times per day! But they're the same guys who have no life outside of their training and don't accept that 'normal people' have to go to work and run a household. So my advice is roll as often as you can – with the goal being twice a day for each hot spot. The good news is that to do this you don't need to 'warm up' or be wearing any special exercise clothing, nor do you have to necessarily do all the hot spots at once, so you can spread their treatment throughout the day if that helps – just do your best. This section can be continued until you feel that you have had a positive effect on the hot spots – that could mean 4–6 weeks of constant work. However, there is a 'but' coming ... this time frame may be ambitious if you are simultaneously doing a significant amount of running or intense weight training as you will, in effect, be constantly 'heating' up those hot spots. Don't be despondent though. Just remember what I said earlier about cleaning your teeth – if you miss one session, you might not notice, but if you miss a few then you will; conversely, if you clean them but also grind them all the time, all the brushing in the world can't repair the damage. So, if you truly want to get on top of the hot spots, you may need to modify your other activities to give the tissue transformation a chance.

Once you have eliminated or reduced the pain you experience rolling your hot spots (trigger points) to a low level of discomfort, you'll then be ready to move on to the next phase: invest and mobilise. This is where we incorporate much larger areas of the body – the good news is you will most likely find that these new areas of the body are less sensitive than the hot spots you started with on day one.

invest time to mobilise and massage with micro and macro rolls

I know it is human nature to think that quicker must be better, but spending time reducing the sensitivity of those hot spots in the previous section will have been time well spent: you will see faster results than if you had bypassed that section. Even if you are an experienced athlete but new to foam rolling, I would class you as a beginner and therefore best served by starting on the 'find it' section, so rewind if you have skipped to this section.

Just as with yoga, a person who consistently uses a foam roller can be described as 'practising' the techniques. At this stage you are ready to roll your entire body, but it's worth still giving the hot spots close attention with the addition of all their closest neighbours (or, as I like to think of them, the muscles that are upstream and downstream from the hot spots).

Hotspots	Surrounding area
Above and below gastrocnemius	The muscles that stream down to the foot and up to the hamstrings
Inwards and down from IT band	The muscles that stream into the glutes, quads and the tibialis anterior (outside of shin)
Above and below piriformis	All the muscles that stream into the lower back plus glutes
Inwards and above quadriceps/hip flexors	The muscles that stream towards the inner thigh and obliques
Outwards and below pectoralis	The muscles that stream into the deltoids and intercostals
Beneath and outwards from erector spinae	The muscles that stream into the glutes and trapezius

finally, monitor and maintain

Congratulations, if you have worked your way through the initial sections, you are now effectively moving into the 'cruise control' phase. This means that the hard work is over and you can hopefully enjoy the rolling sessions rather than endure them. If you have fast forwarded to this point thinking that 'advanced' stuff must be more effective, please rewind. I've come across this approach many times in my career, but in the case of foam rolling you couldn't be more wrong. Starting with the 'monitor and maintain' movements is like putting all the ingredients of a cake in the oven without mixing them together and expecting a cake to appear half an hour later. If you skipped the previous sections, you will only benefit from some of the moves. I would liken a person who takes shortcuts to being similar to a person who smokes, drinks and has a poor diet then takes a multivitamin tablet thinking that popping a pill will somehow counteract all the bad stuff they do to their body ... Are we clear? No shortcuts!

So if you have worked through the previous sections, you should be feeling fantastic and this maintenance phase will be a joy. In this section, the movements (mostly macro roll) actually become much more relaxed. Now, rather than me reeling off a huge list of muscles, just accept that the moves that feature in this section can simply be classed as 'all the other important bits'. There are at least 642 muscles in the human body, but we don't need or have the ability to affect them all with a foam roller. As I can't think of a good reason for rolling the likes of the levator anguli oris (the muscle that curls the mouth to produce a smile) or the occipitofrontalis (the muscle that raises your eyebrow), I'm going to focus on the 174 skeletal muscles that I can visualise the function of and the large areas of fascia that either wrap or are secreted amidst our moveable soft tissue.

2 the portfolio of moves

which moves should I do?

This section contains a portfolio of moves that I have selected from those I use every day with my personal training clients and are based on the principles I explain in the first part of this book. The only moves that have made it into this book are those that deserve to be here – every one of these moves is tried and tested to ensure it gets results. In fact, I have spent hours using them myself and teaching them to my personal training clients or other personal trainers in workshops, who over the years have included men and women from 16 to 86 years old, from size zero through to 280lbs. These clients have, justifiably, only been interested in the moves that work – and that is what you have here in this portfolio.

It is not an exhaustive list of moves, simply because many extra moves that could have been included use the foam roller simply as a 'prop' rather than a tool, or they are really just subtle adaptations of those already included here. I've also excluded any moves which use the foam roller as a balance tool, because frankly there other better products available if that is the goal; you'll find some of these in the 'don't waste your time' section at the end of the portfolio of moves.

presentation of the moves

I wanted to show the moves as a complete portfolio, rather than simply wrapping them up into workouts, because you are then able to see how they relate to each other. Understanding these relationships is something I encourage everyone to do because foam rolling is a very personal activity and as you accumulate experience there is no reason that you can't adapt some of the moves if it enables you to erase pain more effectively.

exercises to avoid

I've included a section for reference of exercises that I don't recommend. Some of these are exercises I have seen in gyms around the world which I think are duplicates of other moves, misguided or unproductive, or achieve little benefit. Personally I like to use products for their primary use, so using foam rollers for strength and conditioning doesn't really add up to me. By doing self myofascial release (SMR), I'm trying to 'relax' and make tissue more malleable and to do that I have to get my brain to accept that the localised pain is a worthwhile payoff for the benefits we are achieving. However, I can't seem to achieve that same acceptance when doing some of the conditioning exercises I've seen and tried on a foam roller – moves like the modified plank, child pose or superman pose seem to be hard for the hell of it, which is an approach that has never really fitted in with my way of thinking. I've tried to explain why I'm not a fan of these moves and to keep things positive, so I've also included a suitable replacement for each of them.

The third part of this book then goes on to present a selection of sessions, designed for a range of purposes (goals), following my method of progressing through erasing pain, investing and maintenance. No doubt some people will jump straight to the training sessions, however, I find understanding the 'why' as well as knowing the 'how' generates better outcomes for most people so refer back to the portfolio of moves if you want the detailed description of how to perform the exercise. Unlike in some of the other books in the series where you are able to go faster or lift heavier weights, there is a finite level of achievement when exercising with a foam roller. When you reach the maintenance phase in this book, you really have achieved a great deal and the best strategy is to keep repeating the maintenance cycle.

every muscle plays a part

Like many other people, when I was first introduced to foam rolling I was under the impression that it was just a case of 'steamrolling' the muscles into submission, i.e. rub it until it doesn't hurt anymore, then move on. Well, although that may be better than doing nothing, the reality is that a slightly more considered approach will get better results. If we simply chase pain around the body, we'll get stuck and only work on the tissues that have reached a critical stage of damage or fatigue. So whilst I don't expect anyone to do every muscle every time, it is important to try and roll out the entire body at least once a week.

key to each move

As you read through the exercises, you will notice that each is identified by the following key words: erase, invest and maintain. A quick glance will also tell you if the move is targeting a hot spot (as a guide these cover an area smaller than the palm of your hand) or if it's a macro move that incorporates multiple muscles and connective tissue. Any time I say 'SMR' it's simply shorthand for what you are doing to your tissues: SMR stands for self myofascial release, which is an all-encompassing description of foam rolling techniques.

I have written the descriptions as if I am talking to you as a client – the key information for each explanation includes:

- the correct body position at the start and finish of the move
- the movement that you are looking to create.

The latter is important because we need to roll the tissue correctly, not just steamroll it.

When I work with my PT clients I avoid over-coaching the movement as my goal is to see them move in a lovely 'fluid' way, where the whole movement blends together.

reps

For the vast majority of the moves I don't say exact numbers of repetitions you should do of each move as it will very much depend upon your own personal tolerance level to 'pain', and also your own needs.

tempo

Moving at the right speed when you roll is essential. If you are receiving a sports massage, you have no control over how fast the therapist moves over an area with their hands; if they want to go slow because they can feel 'congestion' under the skin, then they will. However, when you are rolling your own muscle and come across the same congestion, you are likely to instinctively rush away from the pain – you need to fight that temptation and go slow. This means taking at least 3 seconds to get from A to B on a hot spot and much longer on the bigger macro moves (those that target multiple muscles in one swoop).

tricks of the trade

For each exercise, I have included a 'tricks of the trade' box which contains a nugget of information that I use to help my clients get the most from each exercise. This might be a physical trick or a coping strategy that helps them get the best out of the move.

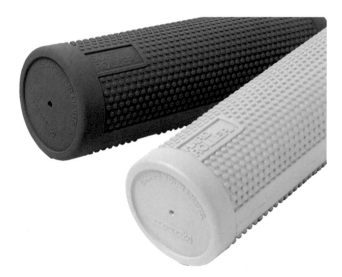

erase pain moves (hot spots)

exercise 1 quads & hip flexors roll (at the pelvis)

● erase ● maintain – hot spot

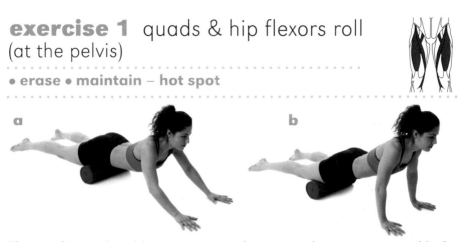

The quadriceps (quads) are your powerhouse muscle group, responsible for forward propulsion, jumping and many other tasks, and are constantly working in conjunction with your hamstrings, so to perform optimally they need to be able to move freely without restriction. That should be a good enough reason for them to have made it in to the hot spot list, but these four muscles have the added complication that one of them (rectus femoris) also flexes the hip, which all adds up to making these muscles extreme multi-taskers and worthy of special attention. The most sensitive spots are normally at the hip rather than the knee.

● Lie face down with the roller underneath you pressing into the front of your thigh just below your hip.
● First roll so that the roller moves up towards your hip until it stops touching muscle and feels like it is only touching your hip/pelvic bone.
● Now switch direction (this movement is generated by your arms and chest) so the roller travels slowly down your quadriceps until it is just slightly above your kneecap (patella).
● Switch direction again and repeat.

tricks of the trade

Once you've done this move a lot, you will find that you can add in a 'corkscrew' action – this means that as you move over the roller you will shift your weight to follow the true route of the muscle rather than working in a dead straight line.

exercise 2 IT band half-weight roll
(outer leg)

• **erase** • **maintain** – **hot spot**

a

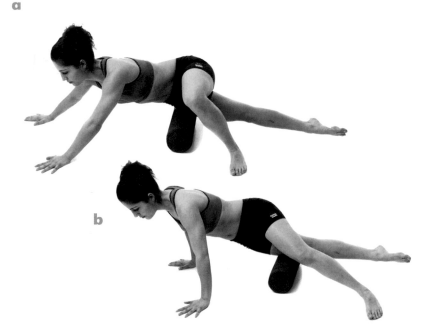

b

Rather than being a specific muscle with an origin and insertion the IT band is an additional component or extension of the tensor fasciae latae. In effect it is an amalgamation of various thick fibres that run down the outside of the leg from the outer hip to the outer knee.

Look carefully at the first picture – there are four contact points: your hands; your outer thigh on the roller; and your foot on the leg that you aren't rolling. For most people this move is doubly difficult as you have to deal with the pressure being placed on your muscles and perform a balancing act, so don't expect it to be perfect first time.

The IT band is always a discussion point amongst trainers and athletes (especially distance runners). For a long time, the most common way of relieving pressure in the IT band after a run or other endurance activity was to cross one leg over the other and push out your hip until you felt a stretch. This feels nice but in reality you are most likely only having an effect upon the ends of the structure rather than benefiting the entire length of tissue – why? Well, it's a slightly simplified explanation, but the IT band doesn't 'slide' against its nearest neighbours, it is stuck to them. With a roller you can be extremely targeted on the spots that are hot and work up and down its entire length.

- Sit sideways on your roller, then rest your upper bodyweight on your hands.
- Bend the non-rolling leg so the lower section is touching the floor, then slightly straighten it so that the roller moves down from your hip towards you knee.
- This may be the most painful of all the moves you do, but try to keep the roller moving super slow so that you get a prolonged period of squeezing against the muscle.
- When you get close to the bony section of the knee, change direction and repeat.

tricks of the trade

If I'm ever asked why use a foam roller, it's easier to have the person try this move rather than try to explain the situation to them. Most people have no idea that they are walking around with so much stored muscle congestion in one area until after they have tried a few reps of this move. Stick with it as the first four reps feel awful, but by the tenth it will be feeling better already.

exercise 3 piriformis roll

• erase • maintain – hot spot

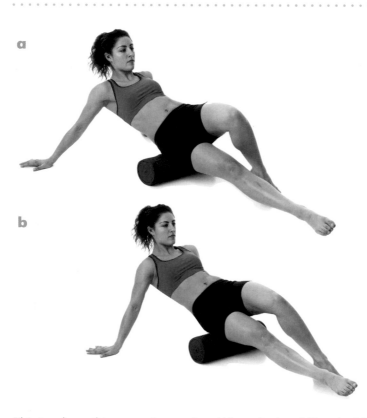

a

b

This is where things get interesting. Where is the piriformis, I hear you say, and why is it such a big deal that it gets on the hot spot list? If you are forced to sit for long periods of time at a desk or driving, the piriformis becomes aggravated due to the forced pelvic tilt that occurs when sitting. There are plenty of muscles that dislike us sitting for long periods of time, but the location of piriformis directly on top of where the sciatic nerve runs through the pelvis gives it the potential to be a real pain in the butt – literally! The piriformis is covered by your gluteus maximus (butt cheek), which is the thickest muscle in most people's body so you have to position yourself in such a way that you get maximum downwards force on the roller while at the same time relaxing the buttock so the effects of the roller not only work on the gluteus maximus but also penetrate all the way through for SMR in the piriformis.

- You can only roll one piriformis at a time. In the picture we are rolling the right side.
- Sitting on the roller with your weight only on your right buttock, bend your left knee and move it over your right leg before shifting your weight back again.
- Rather than sitting at a right angle the roller should be turned about 30 degrees towards the crossed leg.
- Shift your weight forwards until you feel the roller get close to your hip bone then shift your weight the back until you feel the roller get to the crease where your leg and buttock meet.

tricks of the trade

There's no reason to make any of these moves harder than they need to be so if the 'sitting up straight' part is more challenging than the actual rolling, lean yourself against a wall so that all you have to think about is hitting the spot.

exercise 4 gastroc roll
(thick section of calf)

• **erase** • **maintain** – **hot spot**

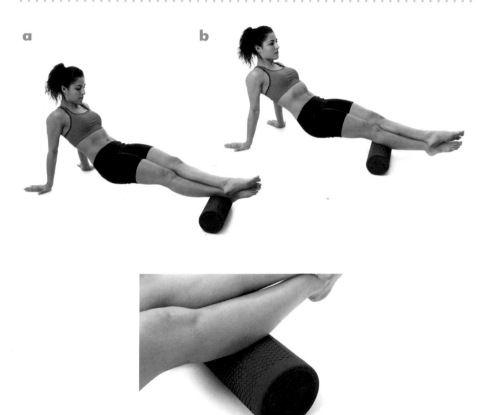

a   b

Many injury niggles begin in the lower leg and force us to adjust our gait (how we walk) to accommodate low levels of pain of restriction. As this is one of the earlier moves pay lots of attention to the information or 'feedback' that your muscle is giving you – it will most likely hurt, but you'll also find it oddly enjoyable as it becomes less painful with each repetition.

● Place the roller at the base of your calf muscle and cross your legs so the other leg is applying downwards pressure on your calf.
● Sit up straight with your hands just behind your hips and lift yourself up.

- Shift your bodyweight so the roller rolls up towards the back of your knee. Make sure you go super slow to ensure the roller has time to do its job.
- When you have covered the length of your calf, reverse the process.

tricks of the trade

This move is transformed if you do it with a 'helper'. This is someone that you really trust as you need them to push down firmly on top of your leg as you roll back and forwards – why? Well, the weight of your own spare leg will be applying about 5–6kg of downwards pressure but your assistant can add approximately 20kg. They could add more if they press really hard but it would be agony so make sure they don't get carried away and stop if you tell them to.

exercise 5 erector spinae roll
(length of spine, straight up the middle)

● erase ● maintain – hot spot

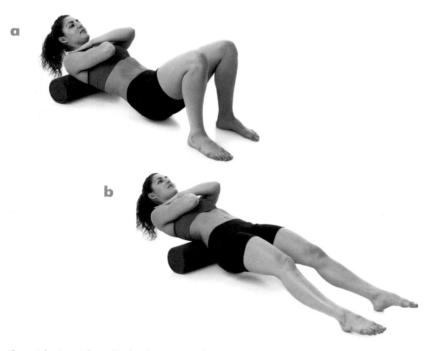

a

b

Considering it's called a hot spot, this might seem like a large area of body to be rolling, but while these hot spots are only as big as the palm of your hand, you may have multiple congested areas spread along the length of each muscle area.

The erector spinae is a long length of muscle and fascia goes all the way from the base of the spine (right down between your buttocks) all the way up to the back of your skull. I don't recommend anyone rolling with their full bodyweight on the roller anywhere past shoulder height because the neck is designed to support vertical loads – not have 60–70 per cent of an adult's weight loaded on to it horizontally!

● Get into position with your hips still on the floor and your knees bent. Place the roller behind your shoulders (not against your neck).
● Cross your arms across your chest – this not only gets them out of the way but also keeps your scapular (shoulder blade) out of the way when the roller passes over it.

- Lift your hips up, then slowly lengthen your legs so that the roller moves down the length of your back until it gets close to your buttocks – if you are very strong, you may get all the way, but being slow and controlled is more important than the distance at this stage.
- Roll back in the other direction super slowly and even pause over any particular hot spots.

tricks of the trade

Foam rolling really is about getting in tune with your body so it's really important to listen to it whilst rolling. Subtle changes to your position, even when inhaling or exhaling, could make the move feel completely different – and whilst what I'm telling is right you may also find that changing your body position slightly could be the difference between it feeling just all right to feeling fantastic.

exercise 6 pecs roll (chest muscle, above breast on women)

● erase ● maintain – hot spot

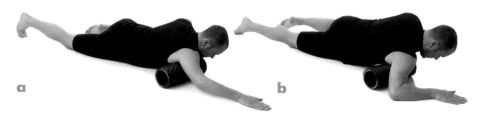

a   b

If you haven't been following a strength programme involving weights, then you may wonder why the pecs (that's pectoralis major and minor, to give them their full names) would be a hot spot. This area of muscle congestion comes not from exertion but from too much time spent with the shoulders rolled forwards rather than retracted; our shoulders start to creep forwards when we sit for long periods of time at a desk, in a car or when doing things like watching TV. Pain from hot spots in this area go hand in hand with the problems we rectified using the previous exercise (erector spinae roll).

I'm particularly focused on getting the roller to work on the minor section of the pecs which lies under the bigger, visable pec major muscle. To do this, we have to get into a rather odd position – but don't be shy, it's worth it.

● You can only roll one side at a time.
● Lie face down and put the end of the roller inside your shoulder.
● Raise your right arm in front of you with the elbow bent to a right angle.
● I find it easier to push forwards by having my left knee bent – you should feel the hot spot almost instantly. When you do, move slowly forwards and backwards over it.

> ### tricks of the trade
> I often see the pecs being rolled sideways rather than my way, which is up and down. I do it this way because I'm trying to 'open' your chest by getting deep onto the strap of the muscle (pec minor), which can pull the shoulder forward if neglected. If vanity is the goal, then neglecting this area is disastrous as the result is round shoulders, which looks awful, no matter how good your pecs are. When you reach exercise 27, we will give the entire chest area some attention.

invest time to mobilise

From this point onwards the moves start to roll larger areas of the body but with particular focus on the direction that key muscles point within our body. All the movements (macro rolls) are performed slowly, taking at least three seconds to go from end to end of short muscles and even longer for the largest muscles.

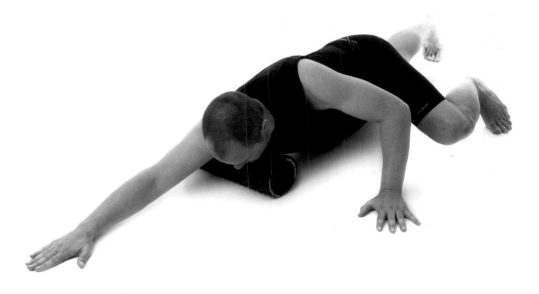

exercise 7 centre of quads (vastus medialis) roll

● **erase** ● **invest** ● **maintain** – **macro**

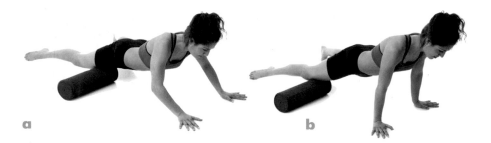

a   b

Your quads are a team, and all four quad muscles play a part in stabilising your knees. The vastus medialis muscle in particular takes a constant beating. The vastus medialis attaches to the femur (thigh bone) on the inside of the groin then at its other end attaches again to the femur just above the inside of the knee. While it can generate a huge amount of explosive force it also keeps the knee joint from being overwhelmed by the even more powerful rectus femoris.

Give this one some extra time if you feel it is as 'hot' as the areas covered in the trigger points section.

● Lay over the top of the roller with it turned slightly in towards the midline of your body. It should be in contact with the piece of flesh above and inside your right knee.
● Bend your left leg, then slowly roll forwards and slightly to the right until you feel the roller roll over the top of the muscle and down the other side.
● Reverse the movement. As you roll this muscle across the grain of the muscle fibres from side to side, you will feel a very obvious thud – this feels odd but it is not harmful, so try to keep as much pressure as possible on the muscle.

> ! **tricks of the trade**
> This is another one of the moves that can benefit from a helping hand. If you struggle to support your bodyweight in this rolling position, you may not be able to get as much pressure on the roller as you need to make it effective, so having an extra hand to push down on your straight leg can turn this from a seven on the pain scale right up to a nine or ten.

exercise 8 upper quads roll wrapping around to the hip

• erase • invest • maintain – macro

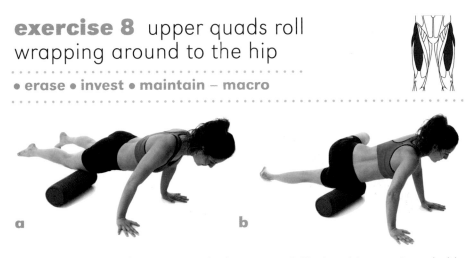

a   b

I warn you now, the first time you do this you won't like it – this move is probably a nine on the 'ouch' scale. It's a double hit of pain because you can't roll this area without getting the IT band in on the act. This move follows the line of the vastus lateralis, which is quadriceps number four if you count from the inside of your leg outwards. It's a muscle that has a hard life because its main roles are to stabilise the knee and also cleverly help to decelerate the knee when it is straightened. Deceleration is a very important skill for a muscle, which is why we always encourage a focus on the concentric and eccentric phases of muscle exercises, rather than just letting gravity take over.

- Lie on top of your foam roller, but with only the top of your right thigh in contact with it.
- Using your hands to help you move, pull your body forwards so the roller moves down your leg towards your knee.
- Try to stay on the outside of your leg, rather than going straight down the midline. This produces a subtle corkscrew motion.
- Slowly reverse the movement and repeat.

> **!** **tricks of the trade**
> Not wishing to state the obvious but breathing is natural and really doesn't need to be coached. However, I often see PTs telling clients when to breathe. Really the best breathing pattern is whatever feels most natural. And remember it may be that in some cases holding the breath is the most natural thing to do – but try to limit this only to the exertion phase of a move.

exercise 9 upper quads roll wrapping inwards to the groin

● **erase** ● **invest** ● **maintain** – **macro**

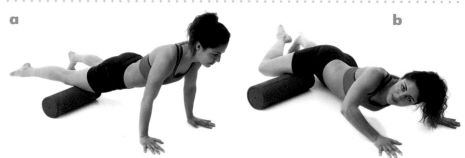

a   b

The good news is that for most people this move is the least painful of the quadriceps exercises. However, if you play any particular sport that uses your inner thigh, unfortunately that might not be the case – with the addition of foam rolling however, you can gradually reduce the sensitivity of this large muscle. If you were counting the quadriceps from the inside outwards, vastus medialis is number one. Like its distant neighbour lateralis, its key role is stabilisation and deceleration of the knee. That means that if you have a job that makes you stay in one position for a long time (driving or standing), you may find that you have particular hot spots down the length of this muscle.

● Lie over the top of your foam roller with just one leg in contact.
● Using your arms, push back so the roller moves up towards your groin.
● It's very easy to avoid the pain (which is counterproductive) so make sure you keep your weight firmly pushing into the roller rather than on the leg that isn't being rolled.
● Try to get the corkscrew action so that when the roller is close to your knee your hips are facing downwards and when it's close to your groin your hip has lifted slightly.

> ## tricks of the trade
>
> For men, there are a couple of things that can 'get in the way' when doing this move. So guys, make sure you adjust yourself before you begin. That's my polite way of making the point that you have to get the roller right up against your crotch to be doing the exercise correctly.

exercise 10 hamstrings roll into your buttock

• **erase** • **invest** • **maintain** – **macro**

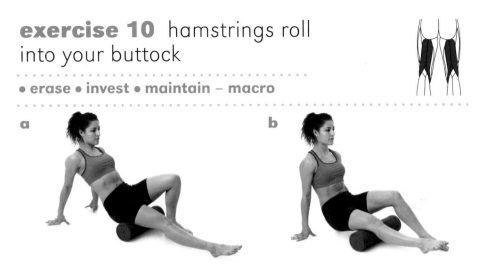

a b

Tight hamstrings are a recipe for disaster for any athlete, especially if your activity requires you to be 'explosive'. What you need to understand about the hamstrings is that, firstly, they have a major influence on your posture because of the way in which they connect to the pelvis and, secondly, they never function in isolation. They always work with their neighbours: your gluteus maximus and your calves.

This is actually a very pleasant exercise to do because it doesn't require you to get into a difficult position and you won't constantly be thinking about how you should be supporting your bodyweight. To a casual observer it looks like we're just sitting on the foam roller – but, of course, we're not. 'Ouch' scale: 4.

- You can roll both right and left legs together but you get a more intense massage if you do one leg at a time.
- Sit with the roller just below where your buttock meets your leg, shift as much weight as you can onto that leg and reach back so that your arms are helping you to keep your balance.
- Roll backwards and when the roller gets halfway down the back of your leg, change direction.
- If you go slightly too far and roll into the buttock, it's not a disaster, but it is better if you can keep focused on just working the hamstring.

> **!**
>
> ### tricks of the trade
>
> If you are in a gym or studio and have access to a plyo box or bench, put the roller on the bench and bend the leg you are rolling, This relaxes the hamstring and intensifies the effect of the roller.

exercise 11 hamstrings roll to behind knee

• **erase** • **invest** • **maintain** – **macro**

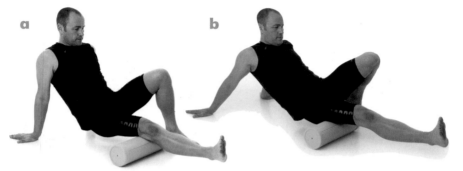

Some clients really want to know how everything works and my job as a personal trainer is to demystify how the body functions. For others they don't care as long as it works, but when we are dealing with foam rolling, perhaps the best approach is to try and visualise how the muscles line up with their neighbours and connect to the skeleton. This move is working on the smaller of the hamstrings and also getting stuck into the lower section of biceps femoris.

- Sit on top of the roller, with pressure on one leg.
- Your starting point is on the outside of the leg that you are rolling, just behind the knee.
- Place your hands behind you for balance and, as you start the movement, push downwards with your arms.
- Your aim is to let the roller move halfway up the back of your thigh, then as you roll back down towards the start position, make sure you have a subtle corkscrew action so you finish at the outside of your knee.

> ### tricks of the trade
> Use the same trick as exercise 10 – put the roller on a bench and bend the leg you are rolling – it feels fantastic. If you have a trusted training partner, then some downwards pressure on the leg you are rolling turns this exercise from seven to an even more effective nine on the 'ouch' scale.

exercise 12 hamstrings roll into your groin

● **erase** ● **invest** ● **maintain** – **macro**

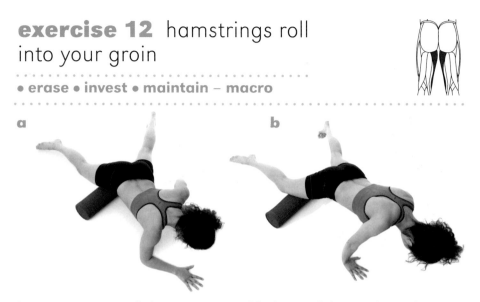

a   b

I am sure most people have an oversimplified view of the muscles in the upper leg: hamstrings, quadriceps and then some little muscles in the inner and outer thighs. However, if you think about the diameter of the average well-developed leg the reality is there are multiple layers of muscles that make up the overall construction of the thigh. This move aims to get directly at one of these deeply buried muscles. It has an extremely long name: semimembranosus (pronounced *sem-ee-mem-brah-no-sus*). Its role is to give us huge amounts of drive through sideways movements, for example a tennis player side-stepping across the court is placing huge demands upon this muscle.

● You can only roll one leg at a time because to get at this muscle you have to open your legs and position the roller as close to your groin as you can get it.
● Shift your hips until the weight is pushing hard into your groin, then with your arms reaching in front of you, pull yourself forwards, keeping your foot parallel to the floor.
● When you get just above your knee, reverse the movement.

tricks of the trade

Wriggle and wiggle! Foam rolling movements generally look 'neat', but to get the roller right into your groin area, it can help to wriggle around so that you ensure the roller makes contact as deeply as possible (where the sun doesn't shine!).

exercise 13 inner thigh roll
(gracilis)

• **erase** • **invest** • **maintain** – **macro**

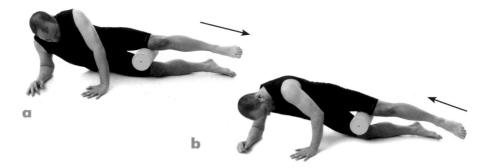

a

b

For everything there is an opposite: hot/cold, light/dark and in the case of the muscle we are rolling here it is the opposite of exercise 2 – the IT band. Without getting too gynaecological, and bearing in mind this relates to men as well, the gracilis muscle goes right up into the groin and around the pelvic floor area. If you put a ball between your knees and squeezed as hard as you can, it is the gracilis that is exerting a lot of that force. Therefore, any activity that requires you to perform powerful lateral movements, such as doing breast stroke legs when swimming, is going to contribute to fatigue and congestion in this area.

This is one exercise you might feel self-conscious about doing if you are in the gym. However, I think it is worth swallowing your pride for the benefits you are going to get.

- Lie on your side and put the roller as high as you can between your legs.
- Let the weight of your top leg push against the roller and shift your hips backwards and forwards 6–8 times, with your bottom leg still. Move it 2cm down the leg and repeat 6–8 times, then move again.

! tricks of the trade

The range of motion that you can achieve in this move is restricted by the amount of mobility in your lower back, which is very limited in this position, so only expect to cover a small amount of tissue at a time.

---

exercise 14 entire length of inner thigh roll (adductors)

● **erase** ● **invest** ● **maintain** – **macro**

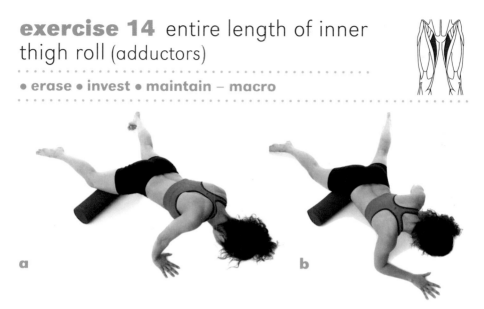

a   b

Unless you have made a concerted effort to train your adductor muscles they are most likely disproportionately weaker when compared to your quadriceps or hamstrings. This is a major issue and leaves you exposed to postural problems and vulnerable to injury. Therefore, it is important to do two things: firstly, strengthen these muscles and, secondly, keep them moving freely. This exercise takes care of the latter.

- Lie on your front with your right leg extended outwards. This should naturally put your foot parallel to the floor.
- Place the roller just above your knee joint and roll outwards so that the roller moves up the inside of your thigh until it makes contact with your groin.
- Without releasing the pressure, shift your bodyweight so the roller moves back down to the start position and repeat.

> **!**
>
> ## tricks of the trade
> Some people seem to make moves like this harder than they need to be. If you push up on your hands (like a press-up), this move becomes really hard, however, I see people do it that way all the time. If you use the technique shown in the pictures, your bodyweight stays on the roller rather than on your hands. The trick here is keeping your chest close to the floor, therefore minimising the weight held with your arms.

65

exercise 15 gluteus minimus roll

• **erase** • **invest** • **maintain** – **macro**

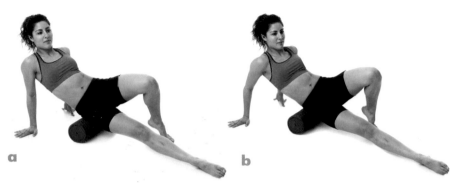

a

b

Our bodies haven't changed a great deal in 100,000 years. However, the way in which we treat them has. Gluteus minimus is a muscle that works hard to make our hips both rotate and adduct (swing the leg outwards). The problem is the gluteus minimus suffers considerably if you sit for long periods of time. This position puts it into a near permanent stretch and this is a problem because overstretched muscles are incapable of exerting their full potential force. I find rolling this area reduces that nagging ache that many people get towards the base of their spine.

Most people's perception of where the gluteus minimus muscle is is incorrect. They view it as being lower down the leg, whereas, in fact, it is entirely above your femur (the longest bone in your leg).

- Lie on your side, with your left knee bent and slightly raised.
- The movement is small and controlled (as if working on a hot spot) as this muscle is at most only the size of your hand.
- Have the roller move only between the bony section of your hips and thigh bone. There is nothing to be achieved by rolling bones.

tricks of the trade

This muscle is much wider at the top than it is at the bottom so it's likely you will feel the roller far more intensely when you roll towards your leg as the fibres become more condensed and compressed. Therefore, take your time and, if necessary, spend longer rolling the narrow end of the muscle.

exercise 16 gluteus medius roll

● erase ● invest ● maintain – macro

a   b

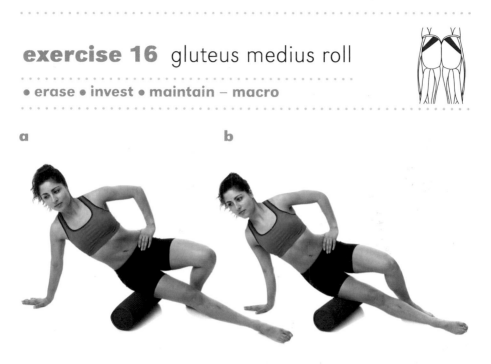

To identify where this muscle is, first place your hand on your buttocks and repeatedly clench your buttocks, then move your hands upwards until you no longer feel you are touching the clenched muscle. You will now be in contact with the gluteus medius. This muscle runs diagonally from the pelvis to your femur (the longest bone in the leg). To roll it, we need to work diagonally.

● Sit on your roller then shuffle forwards until it is only in contact with the very top of your buttock.
● Now shift your hips side to side so that just the portion of muscle above your buttock is being rolled.
● The range of motion is about the size of your hand so roll until you feel you are touching the bone in your pelvis first and then the top of your leg (femur).

tricks of the trade

! Don't make this exercise any harder than it needs to be. Lock out your arm and simply pivot over the foam roller. If you bend your arm, it becomes an endurance exercise and that is not what we are trying to achieve.

exercise 17 gluteus maximus roll

• **erase** • **invest** • **maintain** – **macro**

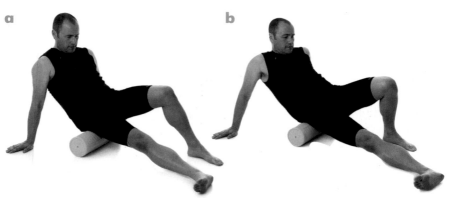

a   b

Gluteus maximus is the densest muscle in the human body for a good reason. It is the power house that helps us run, squat, lunge and jump, and just about any other movement you can think of. So it deserves our attention and certainly benefits from foam rolling. It is important to understand that the left and right buttock are completely separate muscles and that the fibres run diagonally from our centre line. This surprises many people when they start to learn anatomy as they always assume muscles run in straight lines. However, the gluteus maximus is able to develop far more torque by running perpendicular to their muscle neighbours in the spine than they would be able to do if they simply ran vertically.

- You can only roll one buttock muscle at a time so sit on one side of your butt cheeks with the roller at a 45-degree angle to your leg.
- Starting from the top, push backwards with your spare leg until you feel the roller leave your buttock and move onto the hamstrings.
- Reverse the action, but on the return stroke aim to get a corkscrew effect with your hips so that you can be sure you have covered this very large muscle.

> ## tricks of the trade
> Remember it is not simply pressure that causes the good effects of foam rolling – if it was that easy we would all have great buttocks even if we sat on them all day. It's the movement that gives us the benefit. This is a big, wide, deep muscle, so give it the attention it deserves.

exercise 18 pelvis to knee roll
(tensor fasciae latae)

● erase ● invest ● maintain – macro

a   b

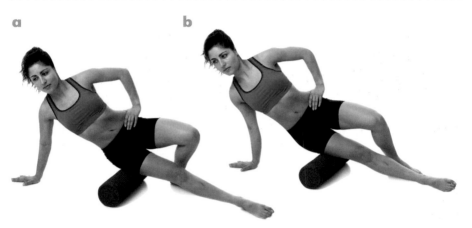

This collection of tissues helps accelerate hip flexion, hip adduction and internal rotation of your hip, so it is an extremely important multi-purpose muscle.

● Lie on your side with the roller above your thigh bone (top of the femur).
● Your top hip needs to be slightly rolled back. This is easiest to achieve by bending your top leg as shown.
● Reach as far away from the roller as you can with your arm.
● Pull with your arm to move your entire body over the roller until it touches the outside of your knee.
● Slowly roll back in the other direction.

> **!** **tricks of the trade**
>
> At approximately the midpoint of this muscle there is a section of thicker tissue so you are likely to feel the most discomfort before and after you roll over this midsection. Left unsupervised, clients often move more quickly over the painful sections. I know it's unpleasant but try to avoid doing this and keep the speed consistent over the movement.

exercise 19 psoas major roll

• erase • invest • maintain – macro

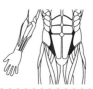

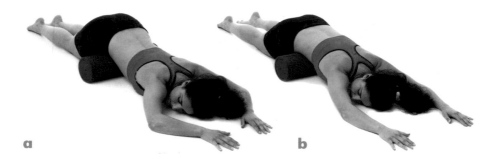

a   b

Psoas (pronounced '*so-us*') is the hidden hero of the abdominals though it's considered the poor relation to rectus abdominus. You always hear people say 'I want to get a six pack', but the reality is a well-conditioned, correctly functioning psoas (the lowest section of the abs) that will contribute to giving you a flat, strong torso as well as providing you with fantastic stability in the lumbo-pelvic region.

- Lie on the roller with it in line with your belly button.
- You must now relax your abdominals, so that your bodyweight is all on the roller.
- Reach your arms forwards, fighting your instincts which are telling you to contract your abdominals and keep them relaxed so that your psoas continues to feel pressure.
- Roll until you get to the pubic bone and reverse the action.

> **!**
>
> ## tricks of the trade
> Many people are sensitive in the abdominal area for reasons other than muscle tissue issues (for example, abdominal bloating, IBS, period pains, etc.), so rolling such a large area at once can be too uncomfortable. Therefore, this is one of the moves I will sometimes perform using a ball, similar in size to an American softball (bigger than a cricket ball) because the surface area/contact point of a ball is smaller so you can target the areas you want to appply pressure.

exercise 20 internal and external obliques roll

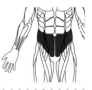

● **erase** ● **invest** ● **maintain** – **macro**

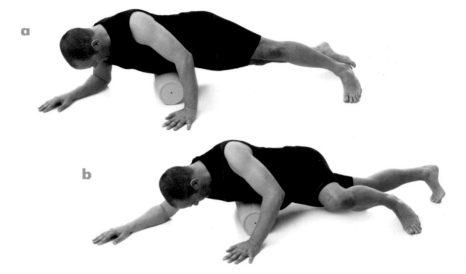

a

b

If you are extremely lean, you will be able to see your internal and external obliques wrapping around your torso from the sides of your six pack and all the way to your lower back. These muscles run at a 45-degree angle, therefore, we are rolling on the bias of our body.

● Lie on your roller at a 45-degree angle, resting on your pelvis.
● Push away with your arms until the roller is touching your ribs.
● Reverse the action.

> **tricks of the trade**
>
> I know that some people like to use the roller as a strength and conditioning tool, however, with moves like this it is far better to be as relaxed as possible, rather than supporting your bodyweight like you would when doing a plank exercise.

71

exercise 21 rectus abdominis roll

● **erase** ● **invest** ● **maintain** – **macro**

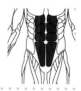

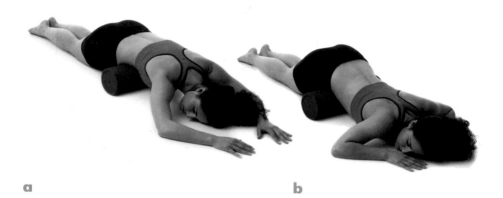

a   b

Prepare to be surprised: the six pack is actually not six muscles, it is one – namely the rectus abdominis. And more surprisingly it isn't one muscle divided into six sections, it is, in fact, divided into eight with the top two sections connecting to your ribs. The definition that so many people aspire to achieve actually depends upon two important criteria: firstly, a very low body fat percentage and, secondly, genetics. This is because the six pack effect relies upon how thick the tendonus material is; it's the width of this division that will give you a more distinct six pack.

● Start with the roller resting on your ribs and relax the abdominal muscle (this means you will need to breathe softly).
● Pull forwards with your arms slowly moving the roller down your abdominal wall until you reach just below your belly button.
● Pause and reverse the action.

> ! **tricks of the trade**
> Unfortunately, dysfunction in the rectus abdominus can actually be self-inflicted: poorly performed crunch sit-ups will cause your abdominals to shorten, giving the person the appearance of having a 'pot belly'. Foam rolling can really alleviate this situation, especially if you rectify the round shoulders that normally accompany this posture.

exercise 22 erector spinae roll

● erase ● invest ● maintain – macro

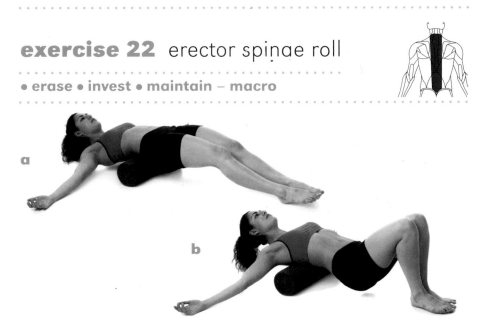

I often record my presentation so I can listen back and hopefully improve my performance. On a recent recording where I was speaking to a group of trainers I said 'scapular retraction' 39 times in one hour. This wasn't because I was supposed to be talking about posture but because the group of PTs in front of me had awful postures. Basically most of them had overtrained their pecs, developing round shoulders and could no longer maintain scapular retraction; clearly they don't practise what I preach! If this is you, then the erector spinae will be stressed and fatigued.

● Lean against the roller so it is much closer to your buttocks than it is your shoulders.
● Let your arms flop backwards to fully expose the muscle that is going to be rolled.
● Push backwards with your legs so that the roller slowly moves up your back until it almost reaches your neck, then reverse the movement.

! tricks of the trade

This move can give instant gratification and relief. There will most likely be hot spots along the length of the muscle, which will heighten the pain factor, so if anyone ever asks for a demo of foam rolling in the gym, this is the move I show them as it always makes a dramatic impression.

exercise 23 multifidus roll

● erase ● invest ● maintain – macro

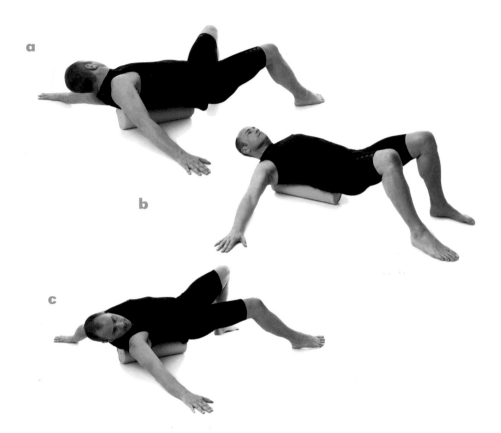

The fibres of this very long muscle actually run from left to right, rather than up/down and therefore can become awfully dysfunctional if you have round shoulders – which makes this move a winner for anyone that spends too much time sat down at a desk or driving.

● Lie on the roller so that it is exactly in the centre of your spine between your shoulders.
● Your weight is spread between your hands touching the floor, your feet and the roller.
● Gently rock from side to side so that you feel the roller working its way between the groove of muscle running the length of your back.

- If you only have a short roller, you will need to move it down towards your hips and repeat the movement to ensure you have rolled the entire length of the multifidus.

tricks of the trade

When working with clients it's good to step back and observe their entire body (many trainers seem to just look at the face but that tells you very little). By looking at the whole body, you can see tension. In this move that's likely to be in the inner thighs so, if the feet are pointing straight up, relax the legs. Alternatively if you're working out on your own be self-aware – acknowledge tensions in your legs and make sure they are relaxed.

With all these weird and wonderful names of muscles, I do hope you are not feeling this book has turned into a lesson in anatomy. The reality is there is 'nice to know' and 'need to know' information, and undoubtedly you could foam roll randomly and achieve some improvement. However, I genuinely believe that by going into the right amount of detail you will have a more holistic understanding of how each one of these moves will benefit you.

exercise 24 rhomboids roll

• erase • invest • maintain – macro

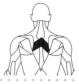

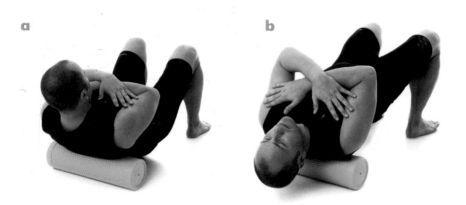

a   b

The rhomboids are another pair of muscles that experience huge amounts of overload if your posture is poor but which can also be quickly rehabilitated.

- Lean against the roller so it is in the centre of your spine.
- Wrap your arms across your torso to fully expose the muscle that is going to be rolled.
- Push backwards with your legs so that the roller slowly moves up your back until it almost reaches the base of your neck, then reverse the movement.

> **!**
>
> ### tricks of the trade
> Don't be surprised if you hear some clicks coming from your spine during this move. Whilst I don't like therapists manipulating bones this is different – it's just your body responding to the pressure – and most importantly there are no sudden movements and your spine is straight rather than rotated as it is when a bone-cracking therapist crunches you.

exercise 25 trapezius roll

● erase ● invest ● maintain – macro

a   b

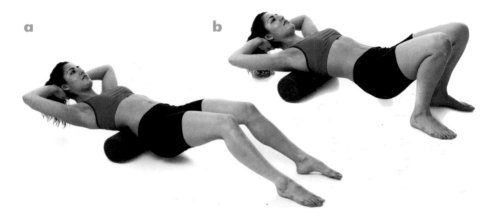

If you want to lift your shoulders up, down, forwards or back, then the trapezius is going to make it happen. It is also the muscle that makes you nod your head when you are asked if foam rolling hurts the first time you do it so frankly it is a muscle with a lot of responsibilities. It doesn't respond to being 'stretched' and one third of its width is a mixture of fascia and tendon, so foam rolling is like a magic wand to this diamond of a muscle.

● Lean against the roller so it is much closer to your buttocks than it is your shoulders.
● Put your hands behind your head and support the weight of your head. This position will fully expose the muscle that is going to be rolled.
● Push backwards with your legs so that the roller slowly moves up your back until it almost reaches your neck, then reverse the movement.

! tricks of the trade

The trapezius goes right up to your skull, but I don't like you rolling the neck with much force so I like to finish off this section of tissue with a slow, smooth massage using my thumbs. Simply start at the base of your neck and slowly rub upwards until you feel your skull.

exercise 26 latisimus dorsi roll

• erase • invest • maintain – macro

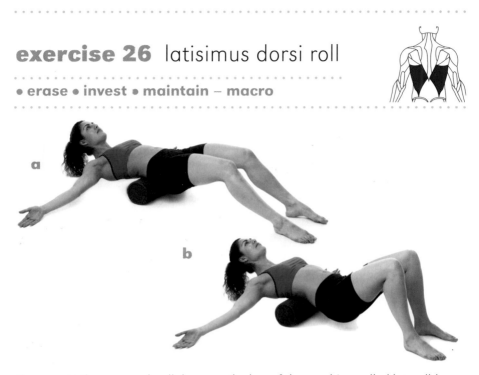

If you go to the gym and pull down on the bar of the machine called lat pulldown, there is very little activity in your lats unless you lean back and have a decent amount of weight on the bar – why? Because this is a massive muscle that wraps around your back like a cape. It has serious amounts of fascia that work with the muscle fibres, which, all in all, makes it a dream to roll because you simply can't miss it.

● Lean against the roller so it is much closer to your buttocks than it is to your shoulders.
● Stretch your arms outwards so they are in a crucifix position. This position will retract your scapular and fully expose the muscle that is going to be rolled.
● Push backwards with your legs so that the roller slowly moves up your back until it almost reaches your shoulder blades, then reverse the movement.

tricks of the trade

Ask most people where this muscle connects and they say 'on the back of the shoulders', but, in fact, it extends all the way under your armpits connecting to the front of the long bone in your arm (humerus).

exercise 27 pecs major roll

• erase • invest • maintain – macro

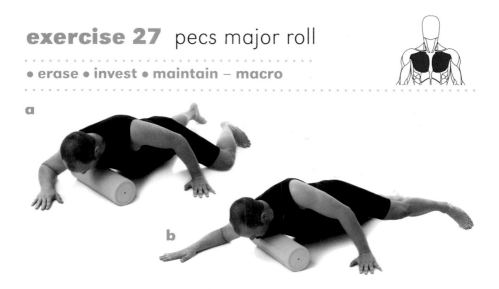

a

b

If you lift weights (especially heavy ones) then this move is essential to help avoid a rounded shoulder posture. Looking around an average gym, the most common example of poor posture you will see is rounded shoulders (in extreme cases this develops in to full blown kyphosis). How can this be the case in a place where everyone is lifting weights in a quest to improve their posture? Well, I think that, especially in the case of men, they overtrain the sections of body that they can see and ignore the bits that are out of sight – so it's their over-attention to the pecs that becomes their downfall in the quest for better posture.

- Put the end of the roller inside your shoulder so that is pointing towards 11 o'clock, then raise your arm in front of you with the elbow bent to a right angle.
- I find it easier to push forwards by having my left knee bent. You should then feel the pressure almost instantly. When you do, move forwards and backwards slowly, working from side to side rather than up and down as we did in exercise 6.
- Repeat on the other side with the roller pointing towards 1 o'clock.

> ## tricks of the trade
> Having never had breasts I bow to the superior knowledge of my female clients on the subject of boobs – they tell me it's the thicker section of muscle along the top of the chest that needs most attention so use the end of the roller to work it and don't go near the actual breast tissue.

exercise 28 triceps roll

• erase • invest • maintain – macro

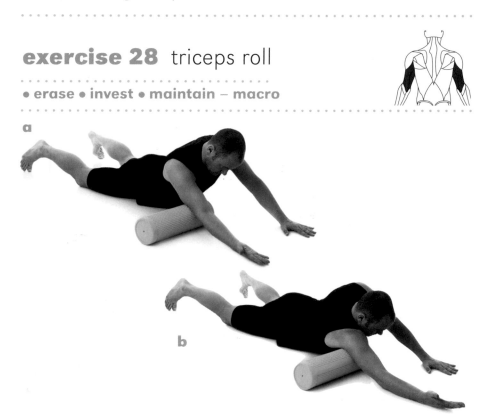

a

b

If you haven't trained them in the last couple of days, then triceps only require a quick roll. However, if you are suffering the after-effects of a training session, this is going to hurt simply because the triceps already ache and they don't have any padding under them so they're getting pressure from both sides (roller on one, bone on the other).

- Lie on your front (but try not to tense your triceps).
- Start at the elbow and roll towards your armpit, applying as much downward pressure as you can tolerate.
- Repeat in the opposite direction.

! tricks of the trade

If you find a hot spot (which is likely to be at one of the two ends), get stuck in with your hands: apply a firm amount of pressure with your index finger on the spot.

exercise 29 biceps roll

● erase ● invest ● maintain – macro

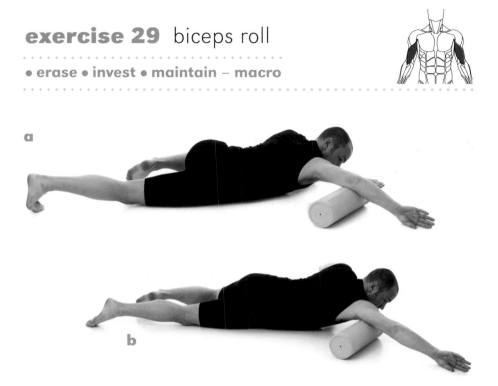

a

b

Considering how much work they do all day I see very few biceps injuries, but they do get fatigued and can exhibit severe delayed onset muscle soreness after a heavy session of weights – so in the interest of treating the body as a whole, this rolling action is dedicated to the 'guns'!

● Drape your arm over the top of the roller and ensure that your thumb is pointing downwards.
● Using your legs to initiate the movement, push forwards and try to ensure the roller is rolled over the entire biceps from elbow to shoulder.
● Repeat the movement in the opposite direction.

tricks of the trade

If you find any particularly hot spots on the biceps, you can try some trigger point work on them by gripping the muscle between your thumb and finger and squeezing hard.

exercise 30 forearm roll

● erase ● invest ● maintain – macro

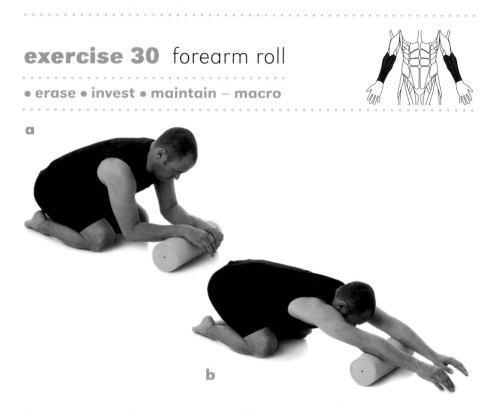

a

b

You have 11 significant muscles that generate movement in your hands and wrist, plus there is fascia and ground substance in abundance in this area, so time spent rolling here is time well spent – especially when you consider every upper body exercise you ever do relies upon these muscles working optimally.

● This move is best performed sat at a table.
● Place the roller infront of you, with your forearms on the roller.
● Starting at the wrist, roll forwards slowly. These muscles connect and travel in multiple directions so try to sense where more or less pressure is required.
● Keep as much downward pressure as you can manage and then reverse the direction of movement.

tricks of the trade

Let your wrist and fingers relax whist rolling the forearm. Any tension in these areas will simply detract from the potential benefits.

monitor and maintain (mostly macro)

Some of these moves will look familiar but the subtle difference is that we are rolling much larger areas of the body with each repetition. You can also roll slightly faster than you have until now unless you feel a hot spot, in which case work back and forth until the sensitivity subsides. You'll note I prefer to talk about time per move rather than repetitions so with these moves your goal is 1 to 2 minutes per targeted section of tissue.

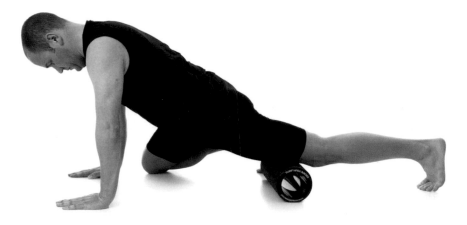

exercise 31 whole back roll

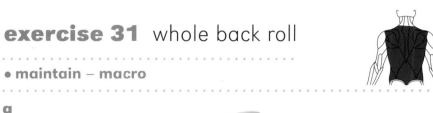

● **maintain – macro**

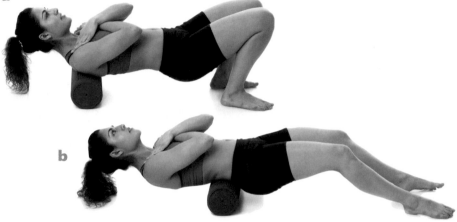

a

b

Prepare to groan! If you are ever asked 'what does foam rolling feel like?', I bet you'll struggle to put it into words other than 'it's great, but it hurts'. This move can, in just a few seconds, make you feel fantastic. I actually have a foam roller next to my desk and whenever I feel the need I'll dive on the floor for a couple of minutes posture break and get stuck in to this move as it is such a fantastic antidote to too much screen time.

● Begin with the roller near the top of your spine and wrap your arms across your chest, bringing your chin towards your chest.
● Push back very slowly with your legs so that the roller moves down your back. You may even feel it going over each vertebra in your spine depending upon how hard your roller is.
● Roll until you feel you are getting near your pelvis, then reverse the movement.

> **!**
> ### tricks of the trade
> Honestly the best advice I can give you from this point onwards is 'don't fight it'. The more relaxed you are the better it will feel.

exercise 32 entire back roll on the bias

• **maintain – macro**

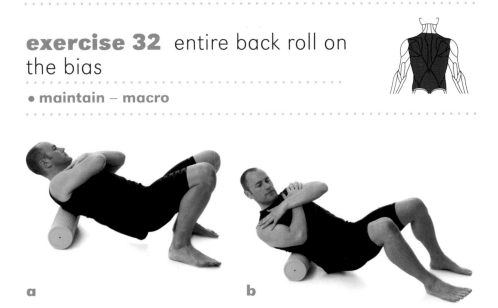

a   b

I like 45cm long foam rollers, as you can roll the entire width of your back and roll around them without it getting in the way if you are supporting your bodyweight through your hands. However, this is one of the moves that can benefit from some extra length – it gives a spectacular deep massage if you can coordinate well enough to start on one side then roll to finish on the other.

● Visually this is similar to exercise 31 but the roller starts and finishes at an angle to your body.
● Begin with the roller at a slight angle near the top of your spine. Cross your arms and bring your chin towards your chest.
● Push back very slowly with your legs so that the roller moves down your back. You may even feel it going over each vertebra in your spine depending upon how hard your roller is.
● Roll until you feel you are getting near your pelvis, then reverse the movement.

tricks of the trade

If you are rolling towards your left shoulder, turn your head to look left, and when going right, look right – the reason this works is that it lets the muscle you are rolling relax.

exercise 33 shoulder merging in to neck roll

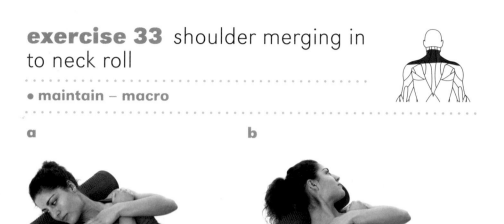

● **maintain – macro**

a

b

Softly, softly is the order of the day with this move. The neck is obviously an area that we need to look after and treat with respect; it doesn't respond well to heavy loads and personally I would never let mine be manipulated by a chiropractor or the like. But it does have a number of muscles and fascia that attaches the head to the rest of the body, so it deserves our attention – just don't feel the need to apply any pressure; the weight of your head is plenty.

● You may find that simply resting your neck on the roller is your limit, which is fine.
● Instead of exerting downwards force by changing body position for this move, we simply turn the head from left to right. This agitates the muscle and fascia without placing excessive pressure on the skeleton.

> ## tricks of the trade
>
> We have tiny little facet joints in our neck, which you can feel under your skin. If you don't get any relief with the roller, put your hands behind your head, lace your fingers together and then with your thumbs gently apply pressure to the muscle running up the back of your neck.

exercise 34 torso front roll

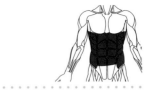

● **maintain – macro**

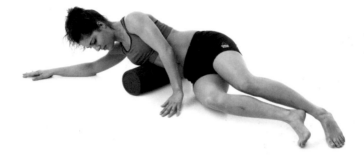

This move is all about getting your ground substance to react and turn into a lovely fluid rather than being stiff and glue-like. Therefore, the direction you roll in is not important as long as you spread around the pressure. It is painful (in that nice foam rolling kind of way).

● Lie on your right side with the roller against your lowest rib.
● Push with your legs and pull with your arms so that you move over each rib one ridge at a time.
● When you get to your armpit, reverse the movement and slowly work your way back down the ribs, preferably taking a slightly different route.

> **!**
>
> ## tricks of the trade
> Holding your breath is not something you are normally told to do during exercise, however, during this move it may help you as it creates a positive intra-abdominal pressure which will help stabilise your torso whilst you roll.

exercise 35 torso seesaw (Russian twist) roll

● **maintain – macro**

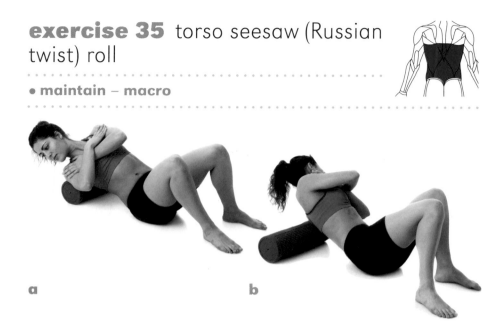

a   b

This is one of my favourite moves from my Gym Ball book and I adapted it for the Suspended Bodyweight Training book, but the reason for doing it here is very different. In those two earlier versions I was working the stabilising muscles but now I'm trying to get pressure into the middle of the latissimus dorsi. You'll know what I mean when you hit the spot.

● Lean against the roller – unlike other Russian twists, this time your buttocks stay on the floor.
● Your body is approximately 30 degrees to the floor and your arms are crossed in front to open the lats.
● Turn to the right. The roller stays still as your body travels along it.
● When you reach the limit of your range of movement, slowly roll back to the centre and repeat on the other side.

> ## tricks of the trade
> Obviously not when personal training but when rolling myself, I find that, because this move can be so painful, doing the move on a bed makes it far more bearable. The softness of the bed means the roller is forced to apply less pressure on the torso as it sinks into the mattress.

exercise 36 loaded inner thigh roll

● **maintain – macro**

a

b

Congratulations, you've reached this far! Clearly you're loving the moves and are probably willing to try everything – which, if you are doing this in public, could be a good thing as this move looks bizarre to uneducated observers. It's worth it though as I don't know a better way of getting at the deep, deep, deep muscles of the groin – apart from letting a sports masseur push their thumbs in very hard.

● You need to be right at the end of the roller.
● Sit upright with the leg being rolled out straight. The other should be bent and tucked in front of you.
● As you move your body so the roller rolls up your leg, you need to corkscrew your hips back and forwards.
● When you reach the top of your leg, roll back down.
● To be effective you need to put as much downward force as you can onto the roller.

tricks of the trade

To make the corkscrew action happen, I think it's easiest to do if, in the 'up' roll, you look at the roller and, on the 'down' roll, you look away from it. This simple head movement will cause your hips to move forwards and backwards in the desired manner.

89

exercise 37 underarm rub roll

● **maintain – macro**

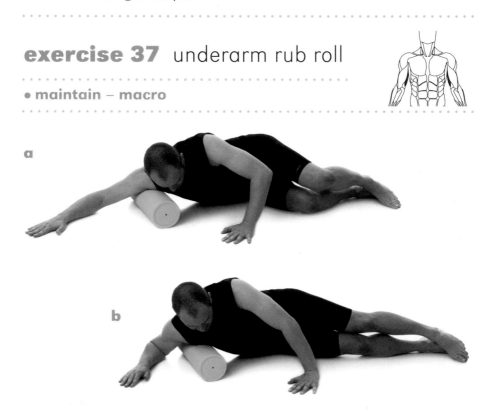

a

b

It's very hard to find this hot spot just by pressing around with your fingers but as soon as you get the roller under your arm, you will hit the spot.

- The best way of describing the starting position is: lie on your side as if reading a book, supporting your head with your hand.
- With the roller in place, straighten your arm and slide you hand away from you so that the roller moves a very small amount under your armpit.
- Keep shifting your weight back and forth across the hot spot.

> ! **tricks of the trade**
> This move is so concentrated that it is best done with no clothing between you and the roller.

exercise 38 sway side to side above centre of gravity (COG) roll

● **maintain – macro**

a   **b**

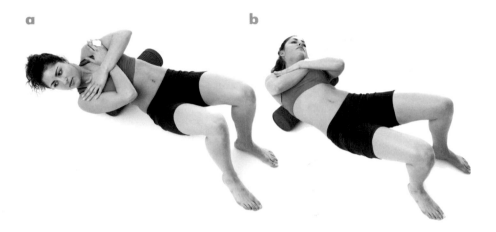

There is a massage technique called 'petrissage' that kneads the muscle tissue under the skin by grabbing and twisting sections of skin and muscle to energise the tissue. This move is a do-it-yourself version of that hand action, with the only difference being you can apply as much pressure on the muscles as you like – unlike when a masseur does it and you are limited by their strength.

● Place the roller in line with your scapular and wrap your arms across your chest.
● Lift your hips off the floor and sway your lower body from side to side.
● The roller should stay in place and you are effectively twisting your skin against the surface of the roller.

! tricks of the trade

This move only hits one spot at a time so if you have the core stability, shift your weight so that you repeat the process over one vertebra at a time moving up and down your spine, swaying on each selected spot at a time.

---

exercise 39 sway side to side below COG roll

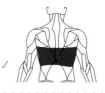

● **maintain – macro**

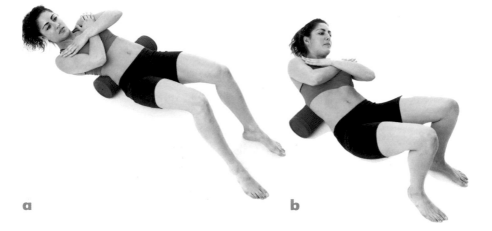

a   b

This move is very similar in description to exercise 38, however, the roller is placed much lower down your back. If you find that the position is uncomfortable, it's a good idea to rest your shoulders on a cushion or, if you have one, a yoga block.

● Place the roller below the curve in your spine and wrap your arms across your chest.
● Lift your hips off the floor and sway your lower body from side to side.
● The roller should stay in place and you are effectively twisting your skin against the surface of the roller.

> **!**
>
> ### tricks of the trade
> Don't use a roller with big ridges for this move – it'll be too painful and you'll tense up.

exercise 40 every vertebra, notch by notch roll

• **maintain – macro**

a

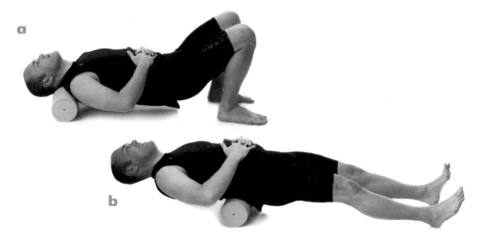

b

Don't do this move until you have worked your way through the less intense positions. To be able to do this well you need to be able to extend your spine and also relax your abdominals at the same time, plus be coordinated enough to push and pull with your legs so the area being rolled stays as relaxed as possible.

- Begin with the roller near the top of your spine. Your head is also near the floor.
- Push back very slowly with your legs so that the roller moves down your back. You may even feel it going over each notch of your vertebra depending upon how hard your roller is.
- Go no further than your pelvis. If it's too difficult to control the movement, stop before you reach that point.

! tricks of the trade

If you have long hair, don't let it get rolled over as it will pull it and really hurt!

---

exercise 41 legs raised, back roll, with flipped chair

● **maintain – macro**

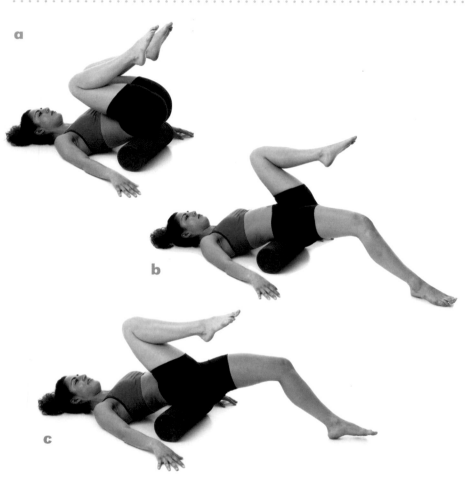

a

b

c

An odd name, buit to me it looks like you've just tipped a chair backwards and ended up on the floor! The lower back is a mass of muscles, ligaments, tendons, fascia and of course plenty of ground substance. We need to apply pressure but not get you in such a position that the intervertebral discs are overly compressed. To overcome this, I find this reclined seated position works great.

- Sit in front of your roller with it tight against your lower back. Making sure it doesn't slip away, slowly lie down so your shoulders are on the ground and your legs in the air.
- Carefully move your legs towards the floor and back towards your chest.
- When you have finished, push the roller away before sitting up unobstructed.

tricks of the trade

If you can't get comfortable, put your roller on top of a cushion and then do the move. It softens the touch points and makes the movement feel more fluid as the cushion absorbs some of the intensity.

exercise 42 intercostal massage roll with inhale and exhale

● **maintain – macro**

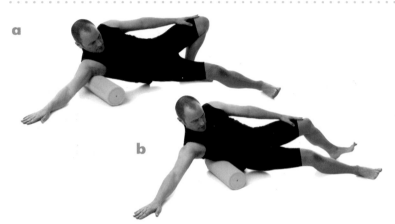

The intercostal muscles fill the space between each rib and are responsible for the stability of the ribcage; they are also intrinsic to the breathing mechanism. We have two layers of this muscle – called internal and external, which run in opposite directions to each other (up and down, left to right). The purpose of this rolling move is not to get at the actual muscle tissue (most of that is inaccessible because of your ribs), so what we are working on here are the many layers of fascia and ground substance that fill in the grooves and junctions around the muscle and ribs.

● Lie on your side with the roller under your arm.
● Move so that you feel the roller bridge itself between two ribs, then inhale fully and slowly exhale.
● If you want to create an even deeper 'massage', gently rock back and forwards on the roller as you take the deep breaths.

> ### tricks of the trade
> Towards the end of each rib there is an area of rib cartilage; sometimes when playing full contact sports, these can become displaced. I know from experience how painful this can be! For this reason, this move is always performed in a slow, controlled fashion – so don't dive or drop onto the roller!

exercise 43 loaded shin roll

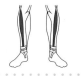

● **maintain – macro**

a   b

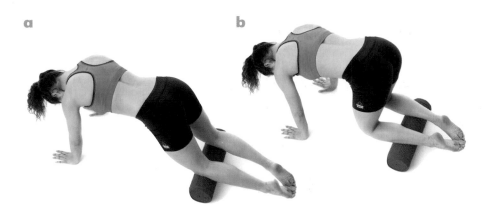

If your calves are tight, your shins will be equally congested. One of the first body parts you learn to massage when you train as a therapist is the shins because it is relatively easy to follow the line of the muscle and feel where it interacts with the shin bone. Of course, what we are interested in is getting the fascia and ground substance to respond positively to our attention and become more malleable.

● To get the maximum downward force on to your shin, you need to kneel on the roller but also keep your hands as close as possible to it so that your body is compact rather than stretched out in a press-up position.
● Turn your big toes towards each other, then let the roller roll down towards your ankle. You need to keep the maximum weight on the roller rather than supporting your weight through your arms.
● When you reach your ankles, reverse the movement.

> **!**
>
> ### tricks of the trade
>
> Some people will do this move and it will be a nice kind of agony, while others will wonder what all the fuss is about. If you experience a lot of pain, persevere with it and be grateful that you are in control – if you were in the hands of a sports masseur, they would most likely keep rubbing no matter how much you complained.

exercise 44 loaded outer calf roll

● **maintain – macro**

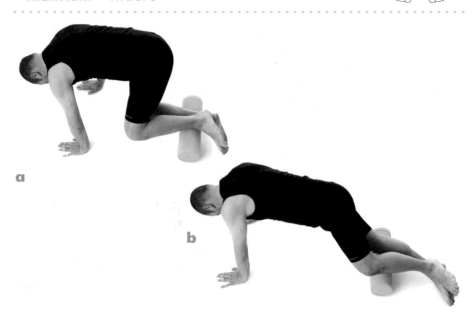

a

b

This exercise is very similar in appearance to move 43 only this time you will be targeting the layer of muscle and fascia on the outside of the leg rather than straight up the middle. The muscles in this space are actually thick so potentially there is more benefit to this move than the previous one. However, I like to think of all these moves as a team rather than individuals, so try to invest some time on the worst areas but also ensure you roll the spaces that feel fine.

● Start in the same position as move 43, then drop your hips to one side before you start moving the roller. You still have both shins on the roller but one is getting far more downward pressure than the other.
● Roll one side for 1 to 2 minutes, then change sides.

> ## tricks of the trade
> In my youth, I, like many inexperienced runners, had shin splints. It is extremely painful and I feel if I had known about foam rolling back then I could have avoided all of the lost training time and excruciating pain. This move along the roller could be the best investment you ever make.

exercise 45 loaded IT band roll

● **maintain – macro**

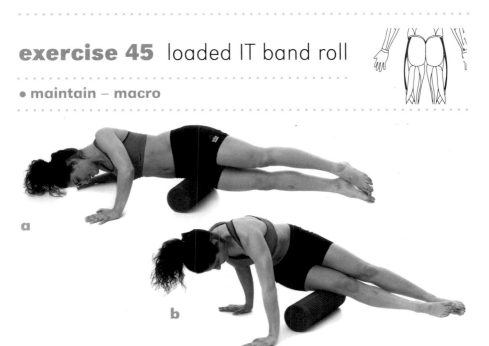

a

b

Spot the difference! This move looks very similar to exercise 2 except even more of your weight is on the IT Band. If we had started with this version, the chances are you would have thrown the roller into the nearest cupboard and never touched it again – but by now you should be ready for the maximum 'ouch' factor that this move elicits. Remember our opinion is changing about how effective 'stretching' the IT band is, so this is your very best option for keeping the muscle and fascia in its optimum condition.

● Your weight is spread between just two contact points: your elbow and the roller. The hand in front is simply helping you to balance.
● Both legs are almost straight as you make your body move over the roller by pushing and pulling with the arm that's touching the ground.
● As you roll in each direction, try to create a subtle corkscrew action with your hips so that you cover the entire outside of your thigh.

> ! **tricks of the trade**
> If you can do this move on one side for 1 minute, well done. If you can do it for 2, then give yourself a gold star and a pat on the back as I can only do 2 minutes if I have an audience!

exercise 46 super soleus roll

● **maintain – macro**

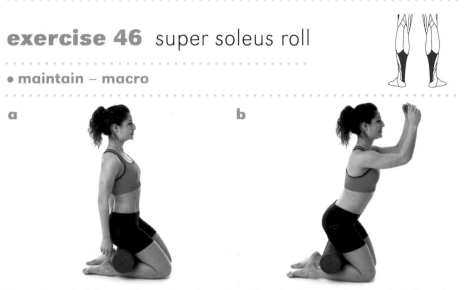

a   b

If you have bulging calf muscles, then the soleus is the muscle directly below the bulge. It actually continues upwards and under the big muscle (gastrocnemius) and also lies behind the Achilles tendon, so it has to work hard in an extremely congested area. It is notorious for becoming tight in people who stand still for long periods of time, with hairdressers being the classic victims. This leads it to being described as a postural muscle but, if you scored well in the movement screen at the start of this book, you'll know it is also a muscle that can be called upon to work during dynamic moves like squats as well as keeping you balanced when you are stationary.

● Kneel on the ground and sit lightly on the roller as shown, just below the more prominent bulging part of your calf muscle (gastrocnemius).
● Lift your weight off the roller, then reapply it so the roller is compressing the muscle it is touching.
● Very smoothly apply and release the pressure on the lower section of your calf muscle before moving it lower down the back of your leg with your hands.
● You only need to go as high as the bulky part of your calf muscle and no lower than your ankle.

---

tricks of the trade

I have a great move for the soleus that you can do with a partner but on my own I always struggled to get enough downwards pressure on the roller. This is why I created this move for you guys who are working alone.

---

exercise 47 back scratch roll out

• maintain – macro

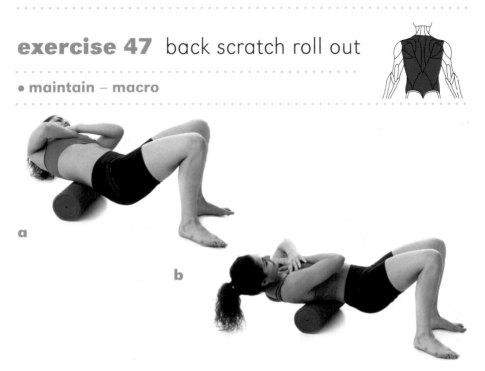

a

b

I'm not sure how to write this without it sounding like a joke but it's now time to go a little crazy! Have you ever seen a bear scratching its back against a tree? I'm sure you have, even if it was just a cartoon. Well, basically, that's the best visualisation I can think of to describe this move. It's all a little random and more vigorous than the previous moves, which look similar.

- Start in a bridge position with the roller in the middle of your back.
- Push with your legs so that your body moves over the roller. By having your arms wrapped around you, you will be increasing your ability to get pressure deep into the muscle fibres.
- At the same time you need to swing your hips from side to side so that your skin and muscles are kneaded and pummeled (that's the bear scratching its back part!). It should feel fantastic.

tricks of the trade

This is another move that benefits from being done with bare skin on the roller as it allows the roller to 'grip' your flesh and really go to work on any adhesions you may have in your soft tissue.

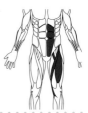

exercise 48 knees to ribs roll and extension

● **maintain – macro**

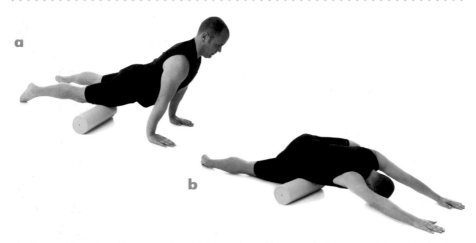

a

b

As I've said earlier I'm not a fan of using the roller as a balance tool for developing core strength, however, while this move requires core stability, the effects of rolling far outweigh any benefits you may be getting in your stabilising muscles. It is a big dramatic movement, which is one of the reasons it features so late in the book, with another being its intensity.

- You can only roll one side at a time (men, if you try and do both together you'll find out why – something gets in the way).
- Start in a plank position with the roller just above your knee and your arms in front of you.
- Pull forward with your arms so that you move over the roll and stop when it gets to your bottom rib.
- Reverse the movement.

> **tricks of the trade**
> If you are really good, you will be able to corkscrew when rolling the leg section of this move, then lie flat when you are passing over the abdominals.

102

exercise 49 foot rocking roll

● **maintain – macro**

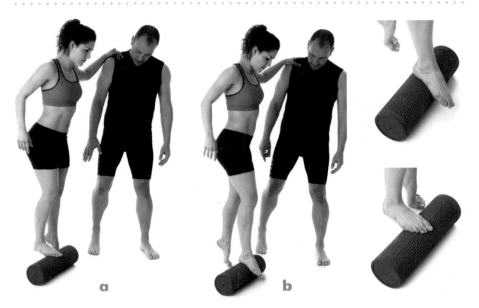

a   b

I may have saved the best until last! This move feels fantastic. If you are ticklish, this could give you the giggles – but, as much as this move gets stuck into the layers of muscle and fascia in the feet, it also feels fantastic in the calves, skin and all around your ankles.

● Place your roller near a wall for balance or work with a partner.
● Stand on the roller and carefully rock back and forwards so that the roller moves from the front to back of your foot.
● After each couple of repetitions, slightly adjust the angle of your ankle so that you are applying pressure on a different section of your foot.

> ## tricks of the trade
> You can perform a more brutal foot massage if you stand on a hard ball then apply pressure against the arch of your foot . This really hurts and some people like the pain. For me, however, the foot rocking shown in the pictures feels so good I would do it just for fun.

don't waste your time

Here are a few moves I see frequently performed in gyms that I think either miss the point of what we are trying to achieve with rollers or are better served if they are swapped for an alternative exercise which can achieve better results.

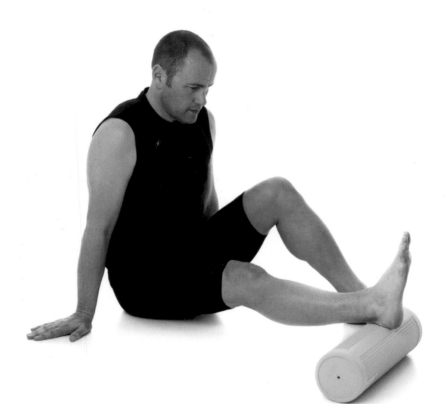

🗑 exercise 50 dead bug balance

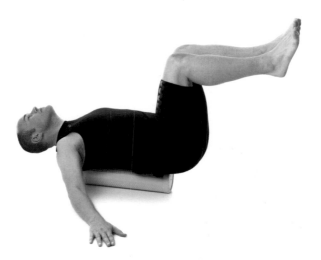

Why not? There is too much tension in the body caused by trying to balance for the roller to have any positive effect.

tricks of the trade

Do the back scratch roll out (exercise 47, page 101) instead.

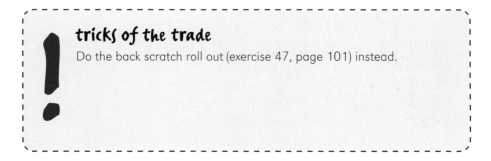

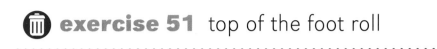

🗑 **exercise 51** top of the foot roll

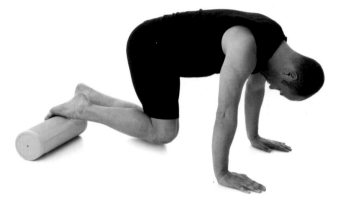

Why not? The top of your foot is predominantly skin and bone so there is nothing to roll that we can affect.

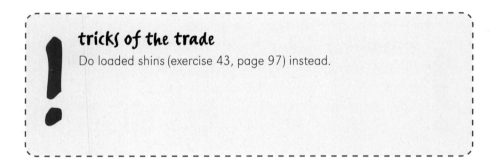

tricks of the trade

Do loaded shins (exercise 43, page 97) instead.

🗑 **exercise 52** roll on top inner thigh

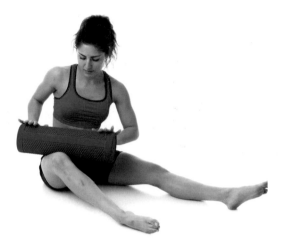

Why not? You simply cannot get enough downwards pressure on the roller to have any effect.

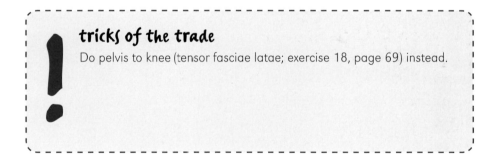

! tricks of the trade

Do pelvis to knee (tensor fasciae latae; exercise 18, page 69) instead.

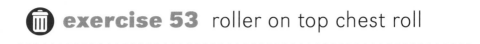

🗑 **exercise 53** roller on top chest roll

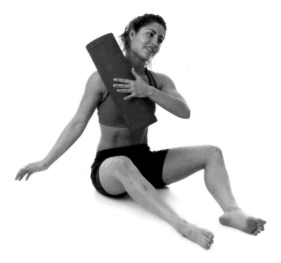

Why not? For the same reason as for exercise 52, you simply cannot get enough pressure on the roller to affect this deep, dense muscle.

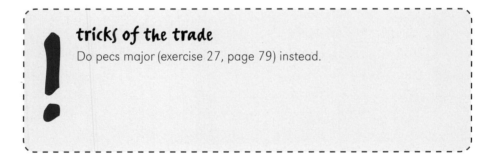

tricks of the trade

Do pecs major (exercise 27, page 79) instead.

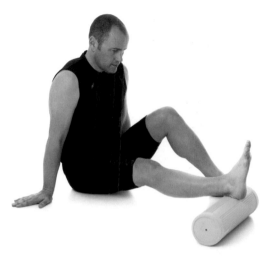 exercise 54 Achilles rub

Why not? Because your tendon has a poor blood supply and doesn't respond in the same way to rolling as fascia does.

! tricks of the trade
Do super soleus (exercise 46, page 100) instead.

3 foam roller workout

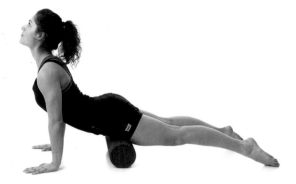

targeted and total sessions

Foam rolling will give you great rewards if you put the work in. Fortunately you don't need to dedicate huge amounts of time to get such results. 20 minutes should be the longest amount of time you need to roll for in any one session. If you don't have that much time, it is okay to do less; you'll still see an improvement but the changes will be slower.

Start with the hot spot programme opposite. Ideally you would roll every day, but if you make time for it for a minimum of three days per week for one month you will still feel improvements. Then, if you feel you have reduced the sensitivity of all your hot spots move on to the next set of programmes. After a similar amount of time you may be ready to move on to the final maintenance sets. However this will vary depending upon what condition you were in when you started rolling and how often you do it each week, plus if you participate in a high volume of endurance-based exercise you may find it takes you longer to reduce your hot spots – but persevere, it's worth the effort.

hot spot programme

Perform each move for 1–2 minutes. Moves marked L + R require you to do 1–2 minutes on the left hand side of body and then repeat the move on the right.

Order in which to do moves	Technique
exercise 1 quads and hip flexors roll (page 47) L + R	
exercise 2 IT band half-weight roll (page 48); L + R	
exercise 3 piriformis roll (page 50); L + R	
exercise 4 gastroc roll (page 52); L + R	
exercise 5 erector spinae (length of spine, straight up the middle) roll (page 54); L + R	

exercise 6 pecs (chest muscle, above breast on women) roll (page 56); L + R	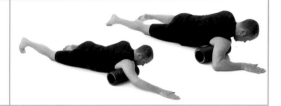

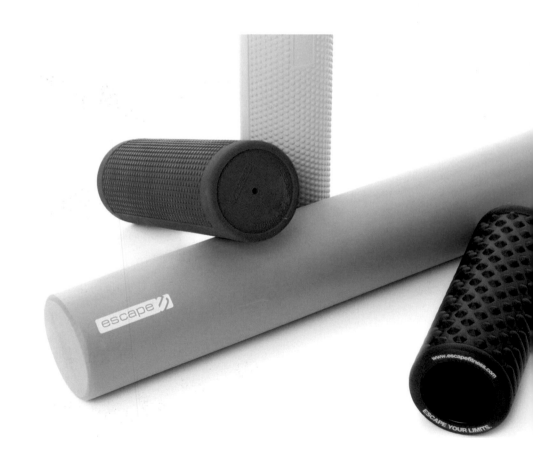

invest and mobilise – total sessions

Programmes A, B, C and D incorporate muscles throughout the body. Each exercise is to be performed for 1–2 minutes. Moves marked L + R require you to do 1–2 minutes on the left side of the body and then repeat on the right. Depending upon how frequently you foam roll it is best to rotate which programme you do – so after four sessions you will have completed programmes A, B, C and D. If, as I hope, you roll more than four times a week, repeat A, B, C and D as often as you like.

Programme A	
Order in which to do moves	**Technique**
exercise 7 centre of quads roll (page 58); L + R	
exercise 19 psoas major (page 70)	
exercise 23 multifidus roll (page 74)	
exercise 27 pecs major roll (page 79); L + R	

exercise 11 hamstrings roll to behind knee (page 62); L + R	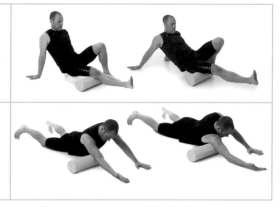
exercise 28 triceps roll (page 80); L + R	

Programme B	
Order in which to do moves	**Technique**
exercise 10 hamstrings roll into your buttock (page 61); L + R	
exercise 8 upper quads roll wrapping around to the hip (page 59); L + R	
exercise 15 gluteus minimus roll (page 66)	
exercise 21 rectus abdominis roll (page 72)	

exercise 22 erector spinae roll (page 73)	
exercise 19 psoas major roll (page 70)	

Programme C	
Order in which to do moves	**Technique**
exercise 9 upper quads roll wrapping inwards to the groin (page 60); L + R	
exercise 14 entire length of inner thigh roll (adductors) (page 65); L + R	
exercise 24 rhomboids roll (page 76)	
exercise 29 biceps roll (page 81); L + R	

exercise 18 pelvis to knee roll (page 69); L + R	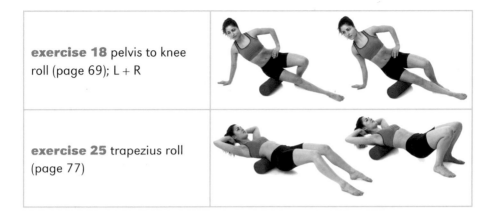
exercise 25 trapezius roll (page 77)	

Programme D	
Order in which to do moves	**Technique**
exercise 13 inner thigh roll (page 64); L + R	
exercise 25 trapezius roll (page 77)	
exercise 17 gluteus maximus roll (page 68); L + R	
exercise 12 hamstrings roll into groin (page 63); L + R	

exercise 16 gluteus medius roll (page 67); L + R	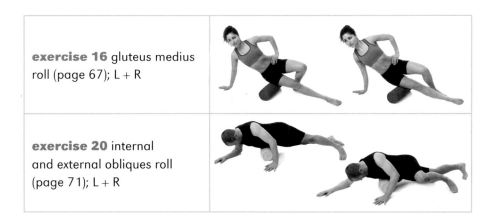
exercise 20 internal and external obliques roll (page 71); L + R	

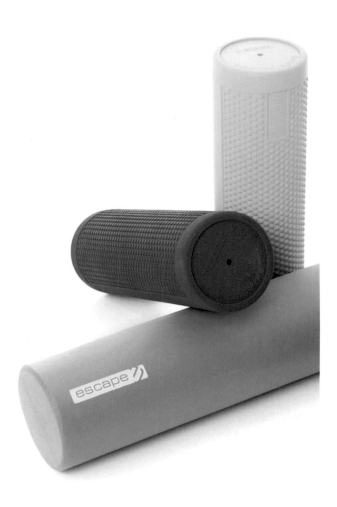

monitor and maintain

Do programmes E, F, G or H to maintain a feeling of mobility and muscle wellness. However, it is best to avoid doing the same programme over and over again, so mix them up to make sure you're covering your entire system of soft tissue.

Programme E	
Order in which to do moves	**Technique**
exercise 31 whole back roll (page 84)	
exercise 35 torso seesaw roll (page 88)	
exercise 43 loaded shins roll (page 97); L + R together	
exercise 37 underarm rub roll (page 90); L + R	

exercise 41 legs raised, back roll with flipped chair (page 94)	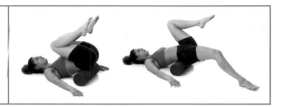

Programme F	
Order in which to do moves	**Technique**
exercise 32 entire back roll on the bias (page 85); each way	
exercise 48 knees to ribs roll and extension (page 102); L + R	
exercise 40 every vertebra, notch by notch, roll (page 93)	
exercise 45 loaded IT Band roll (page 99)	

Programme G	
Order in which to do moves	**Technique**
exercise 42 intercostal massage roll with inhale and exhale (page 96); L + R	
exercise 46 super soleus roll (page 100); L + R	
exercise 38 sway side to side above COG roll (page 91)	
exercise 44 loaded outer calf roll (page 98); L + R	
exercise 34 torso front roll around to the ribs under arm (page 87); L+ R	

Programme H	
Order in which to do moves	**Technique**
exercise 39 sway side to side below COG roll (page 92); L + R	
exercise 47 back scratch roll out (page 101)	
exercise 36 loaded inner thigh roll (page 89); L + R	
exercise 33 shoulder merging in to neck roll (page 86)	
exercise 49 foot rocking roll (page 103); L + R together	

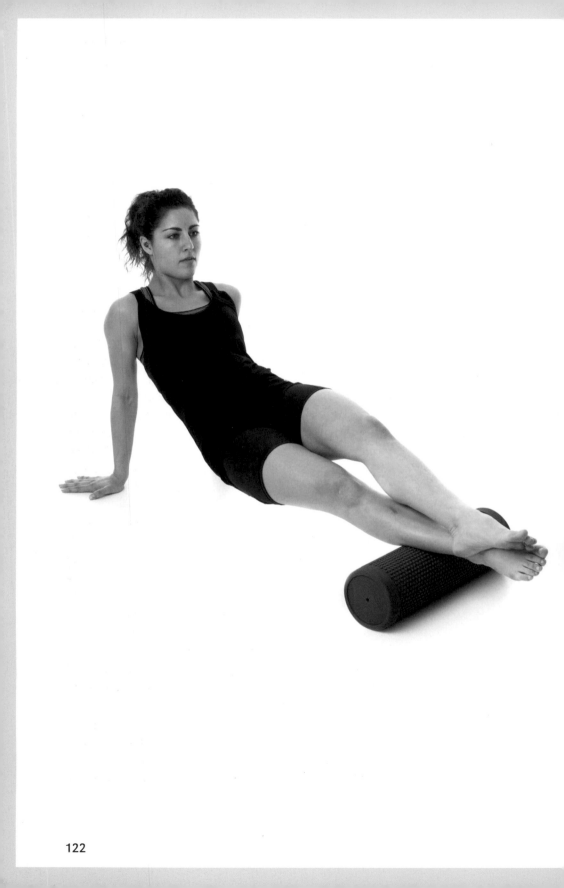

And finally...

The fantastic fitness industry that I work in is still very young, yet it has carved out many niches. There are some people who only ever go to the gym and others who get their exercise hit exclusively in the health club studio, but no matter how or where you work your muscles, foam rolling will not only prove beneficial, but by not conflicting with your chosen method of moving and improving, it will most likely enhance your enjoyment of exercise 24/7. Quite simply this 'therapy' complements everything and competes with nothing. The possibilities are endless: foam rolling is one of the few activities that I can think of that is equally beneficial to fitness novices as to high performance athletes.

Whether you are a personal trainer, sportsperson or fitness enthusiast, I hope you are now far better informed about how to get the most out of the valuable time you spend using your foam roller. All I ask is that you use all the information I have given you in this book and make it part of an integrated health and fitness-driven lifestyle. You may even be tempted to integrate additional equipment into your exercise schedule, like dumbbells, gym balls, kettlebells and suspended bodyweight training, which I've covered in the other books in the Total Workout series. If you do, I know from experience that the benefits from doing so will be even greater now that you are armed with all this information on looking after soft tissue.

As a personal trainer I know that I have a greater than average interest in the human body and the effects of exercise, partly because it is my passion and partly because it is my job. I also recognise that in the busy world we live in, expecting the same level of interest and dedication from clients towards health and exercise is unrealistic, so for me the best personal trainers are those who help clients to integrate exercise into everyday life rather than allow it to dominate. I'm also coming to terms with the fact that as I cruise through my mid-forties everything is a little harder; it seems muscles ache more freely and are harder to maintain than when I was in my twenties and thirties. This 'reality check' of being middle aged has definitely made me a better lecturer and presenter as I can now personally relate so much better to the needs of a wider range of people.

The body is an amazing thing and responds to exercise by adapting and improving the way that it functions. Exercise is not all about pain, challenges and hard work. The fitness industry seems to have come full circle – it started with 'going for the burn' then got all deep and meaningful in the pilates era and has ramped up the intensity again with the vogue for high intensity activity – so it's reassuring to think foam rolling is not a trend but something that will be with us forever. I strongly believe that every minute you invest in exercise pays you back with interest, and that it's all about finding the right balance.

Finding that balance is different for all of us, but I think you can't go far wrong if you train for stability, strength and maybe power. Walk and run, eat healthily and drink water. Find time to relax and stretch/roll, but above all remember: if you ever find yourself lacking in motivation, the best advice I can give anybody wanting to feel more healthy is that if you're moving, you're improving.

fitness glossary

As a person interested in health and fitness there is no need to sound like you have swallowed a textbook for breakfast. Yes, you need to understand how things work, but I feel there is more skill in being able to explain complicated subjects in simple language rather than simply memorising a textbook. The following glossary sets out to explain the key words and phrases that, for a person interested in the body, are useful to know and that will help you get the most out of this book, especially the training section.

Abdominals The name given to the group of muscles that make up the front of the torso, also known as 'the abs'.

Abduction The opposite of adduction. The term the medical profession uses to describe any movement of a limb away from the midline of the body. So, if you raise your arm up to the side, that would be described as 'abduction of the shoulder'.

Acceleration The opposite of deceleration. The speed at which a movement increases from start to finish. When using weights, accelerating the weight when moving it at a constant speed really adds to the challenge.

Adduction The opposite of abduction. The term the medical profession uses to describe any movement of a limb across the midline of the body. So, if you cross your legs that would be 'adduction of the hip'.

Aerobic The opposite of anaerobic. The word invented in 1968 by Dr Kenneth Cooper to describe the process in our body when we are working 'with oxygen'. While the term is now associated with dance-based exercise to music (ETM), the original aerobic exercises that Cooper measured were cross-country running, skiing, swimming, running, cycling and walking. Generally most people consider activity up to 80 per cent of maximum heart rate (see MHR entry) to be aerobic and beyond that to be anaerobic.

Age The effects of exercise change throughout life. With strength training in particular age will influence the outcome. As you reach approximately the age of 40, maintaining and developing lean muscle mass becomes harder and, in fact, the body starts to lose lean mass as a natural part of the ageing process. This can be combated somewhat with close attention to diet and exercise. At the other end of the scale a sensible approach is required when introducing very young people to training with weights.

Personally I don't like to see children participating in very heavy weight training, as it should not be pursued by boys and girls who are still growing (in terms of bone structure, rather than muscle structure), as excessive loading on prepubescent bones may have an adverse effect. There is very little conclusive research available on this subject, as it would require children to be put through tests that require them to lift very heavy weights in order to assess how much is too much. Newborn babies have over 300 bones and as we grow some bones fuse together leaving an adult with an average of 206 mature bones by age 20.

Agility Your progressive ability to move at speed and change direction while doing so.

Anaerobic The opposite of aerobic. High intensity bursts of cardiovascular activity generally above 80 per cent of MHR. The term literally means 'without oxygen' because when operating at this speed, the body flicks over to the fuel stored in muscles rather than mixing the fuel first with oxygen, which is what happens during aerobic activity.

Anaerobic threshold The point at which the body cannot clear lactic acid fast enough to avoid a build-up in the bloodstream. The delaying of this occurrence is a major characteristic of performance athletes, their frequent high intensity training increases (delays) the point at which this waste product becomes overwhelming.

Assessment I like to say that if you don't assess, you guess, so before embarking on any exercise regime you should assess your health and fitness levels in a number of areas, which can include flexibility, range of motion, strength or any of the cardiac outputs that can be measured at home or in the laboratory.

Biceps The muscle at the front of the arm. It makes up about one-third of the entire diameter of the upper arm with the triceps forming the other two-thirds.

Blood pressure When the heart contracts and squirts out blood the pressure on the walls of the blood vessels is the blood pressure. It is expressed as a fraction, for example 130/80. The 130 (systolic) is the high point of the pressure being exerted on the tubes and the 80 (diastolic) is the lower amount of pressure between the main pulses.

Cardiovascular system (CV) This is the superhighway around the body. Heart, lungs and blood vessels transport and deliver the essentials of life: oxygen, energy, nutrients. Having delivered all this good stuff it then removes the rubbish by transporting away the waste products from the complex structure of muscle tissue.

Centre line This is an imaginary line that runs down the centre of the body from the chin to a point through the ribs, pelvis, right down to the floor.

Circuit A list of exercises can be described as a circuit. If you see '2 circuits' stated on a programme, it means you are expected to work through that list of exercises twice.

Concentric contraction The opposite of eccentric contraction. If this word isn't familiar to you, just think 'contract', as in to get smaller/shorter.

A concentric contraction is when a muscle shortens under tension. For example, when you lift a cup towards your mouth you produce a concentric contraction of the biceps (don't make the mistake of thinking that when you lower the cup it's a concentric contraction of the opposite muscle, i.e. the triceps, as it isn't … it's an eccentric movement of the biceps).

Contact points The parts of the body that are touching the foam roller or floor. The smaller the contact points, e.g. heels rather than entire foot, the greater the balance and stabilisation requirements of an exercise.

Core Ah, the core. Ask 10 trainers to describe the core and you will get 10 different answers. To me it is the obvious muscles of the abdominals, the lower back, etc., but it is also the smaller deep muscles and connective tissue that provide stability and strength to the individual. Muscles such as the glutes, hamstrings and, most importantly, the pelvic floor are often forgotten as playing a key role in the core. When I am doing a demonstration of core muscle activation, the way I sum up the core is that the majority of movements that require stability are in some way using all of the muscles that connect between the nipples and the knees.

Creatine An amino acid created naturally in your body. Every time you perform any intense exercise, e.g. weight training, your body uses creatine as a source of energy. The body has the ability to store more creatine than it produces, so taking it as a supplement would allow you to train for longer at high intensity. Consuming creatine is only productive when combined with high intensity training and, therefore, is not especially relevant until you start to train for power.

Crossfit® A multi-level business and training method which uses a holistic approach to exercise and nutrition – these are presented as a WOD (workout of the day) and incorporate influences from weight lifting, sport, metabolic conditioning and gymnastics. Individuals can also participate in Crossfit games® as a competitive sport.

Cross-training An excellent approach to fitness training where you use a variety of methods to improve your fitness rather than just one. Cross-training is now used by athletes and sportspeople to reduce injury levels, as it ensures that you have a balanced amount of cardio, strength and flexibility in a schedule.

Deceleration The opposite of acceleration. It is the decrease in velocity of an object. If you consider that injuries in sportspeople more often occur during the deceleration phase rather than the acceleration phase of their activity (for example, a sprinter pulling up at the end of the race, rather than when they push out of the starting blocks), you will focus particularly on this phase of all the moves in this book. Power moves especially call for you to control the 'slowing down' part of the move, which requires as much skill as it does to generate the speed in the first place.

Delayed onset muscle soreness (DOMS) This is that unpleasant muscle soreness that you get after starting a new kind of activity or when you have worked harder than normal. It was once thought that the soreness was caused by lactic acid becoming 'trapped' in the muscle after a workout, but we now realise that this is simply not the case because lactic acid doesn't hang around – it is continuously moved and metabolised. The pain is far more likely to be caused by a mass of tiny little muscle tears. It's not a cure, but foam rolling or some light exercise will often ease the pain because this increases the flow of blood and nutrients to the damaged muscle tissue.

Deltoid A set of three muscles that sit on top of your shoulders.

Dynamometer A little gadget used to measure strength by squeezing a handheld device that then measures the force of your grip.

Eccentric contraction The opposite of concentric contraction. The technical term for when a muscle is lengthening under tension. An easy example to remember is the lowering of a dumbbell during a biceps curl, which is described as an eccentric contraction of the biceps.

Eye line Where you are looking when performing movements. Some movement patterns are significantly altered by correct or incorrect eye line, for example, if the eye line is too high during squats, then the head is lifted and the spine will experience excessive extension.

Fascia Connective tissue that attaches muscles to muscles and enables individual muscle fibres to be bundled together. While not particularly scientific, a good way to visualise fascia is that it performs in a similar way to the skin of a sausage by keeping its contents where it should be.

Flexibility The misconception is that we do flexibility to actually stretch the muscle fibres and make them longer, whereas, in fact, when we stretch effectively it is the individual muscle fibres that end up moving more freely against each other, creating a freer increased range of motion.

Foam rolling As if I need to tell you, foam rolling is a therapy technique that has become mainstream. You use a round length of foam to massage your own muscles (generally you sit or lie on the roller to exert force via your bodyweight). Interestingly, while this has a positive effect on your muscle fibres, it is the fascia that is 'stretched' most. Foam rolling is actually rather painful when you begin, but as you improve, the pain decreases. Often used by athletes as part of their warm-up. Foam rolling is the poor man's equivalent of receiving a fantastic sports massage; it complements everything and conflicts with no other forms of exercise.

Functional training Really all training should be functional as it is the pursuit of methods and movements that benefit you in day-to-day life. Therefore, doing squats are functionally beneficial for your abdominals because they work them in conjunction with other muscles, but sit-ups are not because they don't work the abdominals in a way that relates to many everyday movements.

Gait Usually associated with running and used to describe the way that a runner hits the ground either with the inside, centre or outside of their foot and, specifically, how the foot, ankle and knee joints move. However, this term always relates to how you stand and walk. Mechanical issues that exist below the knee can have a knock-on effect on other joints and muscles throughout the body. Pronation is the name given to the natural inward roll of the ankle which occurs when the heel strikes the ground and the foot flattens out. Supination refers to the opposite outward roll that occurs during the push-off phase of the walking and running movement. A mild amount of pronation and supination is both healthy and necessary to propel the body forward.

Genes As in the hereditary blueprint that you inherited from your parents, rather than the blue denim variety. Genes can influence everything from your hair colour to your predisposition to developing diseases. Clearly there is nothing you can do to influence your genes, so accept that some athletes are born great because they have the odds stacked on their side while others have to train their way to glory.

Gluteus maximus A set of muscles on your bottom, also known as 'the glutes'.

Ground substance An amorphous fluid/gel found between muscles and fascia that responds to movement, pressure and torsion positively by becoming more liquid. Foam rolling changes its consistency from a gel to a fluid – the medical term for this remarkable transformation is thixotropy.

Hamstring A big set of muscles down the back of the thigh. It plays a key role in core stability and needs to be flexible if you are to develop a good squat technique.

Heart rate (HR) Also called 'the pulse'. It is the number of times each minute that your heart contracts. An athlete's HR could be as low as 35 beats per minute (BPM) when resting but can also go up to 250BPM during activity.

HIIT high intensity interval training A form of metabolic enhancing exercise where you alternate between very intensity anaerobic exercise (near 100 per cent maximum) that is immediately followed by a lower intensity (50 per cent) recovery exercise – these highs and low are repeated until near exhaustion. There are no set durations for HIIT sessions and any modality of exercise can be used for HIIT however running and cycling are the most user friendly.

Hot spots For most people the most sensitive areas of your body are described as hot spots. These are spread throughout the body where there is a natural tendency for higher amounts of tension or inflammation, generally they are where a selection of muscles/tendons attach or cross multiple joints. A good way of visualising these hot spots is as a junction where multiple busy roads meet – invariably there will be congestion in that area, due to the volume of traffic. This translates to these spots being amongst the most painful (but productive) areas to foam roll.

Hypertrophy The growth of skeletal muscle. This is what a bodybuilder is constantly trying to do. The number of muscle fibres we have is fixed, so rather than 'growing' new muscles fibres, hypertrophy is the process of increasing the size of the existing fibre. Building muscle is a slow and complex process that requires constant training and a detailed approach to nutrition.

Insertion All muscles are attached to bone or other muscles by tendons or fascia. The end of the muscle that moves during a contraction is the insertion, with the moving end being called the origin. Note that some muscles have more than one origin and insertion.

Integration (compound) The opposite of isolation (see below). Movement that requires more than one joint and muscle to be involved, e.g. a squat.

Isolation The opposite of integration (see above). A movement that requires only one joint and muscle to be involved, e.g. a biceps curl.

Interval training A type of training where you do blocks of high intensity exercise followed by a block of lower intensity (recovery) exercise. The blocks can be time based or marked by distance (in cardio training). Interval training is highly beneficial to both athletes and fitness enthusiasts as it allows them to subject their body to high intensity activity in short achievable bursts.

Intra-abdominal pressure (IAP) An internal force that assists in the stabilisation of the lumber spine. This relates to the collective effects of pressure exerted on the structures of the diaphragm, transversus abdominis, multifidi and the pelvic floor.

Kinesiology The scientific study of the movement of our anatomical structure. It was only in the 1960s with the creation of fixed weight machines that we started to isolate individual muscles and work them one at a time. This is a step backwards in terms of kinesiology because in real life a single muscle rarely works in isolation.

Kinetic chain The series of reactions/forces throughout the nerves, bones, muscles, ligaments and tendons when the body moves or has a force applied against it.

Kyphosis Excessive curvature of the human spine. This can range from being a little bit round shouldered to being in need of corrective surgery.

Lactic acid A by-product of muscle contractions. If lactic acid reaches a level higher than that which the body can quickly clear from the bloodstream, the person has reached their anaerobic threshold. Training at high intensity has the effect of delaying the point at which lactic acid levels cause fatigue.

Latissimus dorsi Two triangular-shaped muscles that run from the top of the neck and spine to the back of the upper arm and all the way into the lower back, also known as 'the lats'.

Ligaments Connective tissues that attach bone to bone or cartilage to bone. They have fewer blood vessels passing through them than muscles, which makes them whiter (they look like gristle) and also slower to heal.

Lordosis Excessive curvature of the lower spine. Mild cases that are diagnosed early can often be resolved through core training and by working on flexibility with exercises best prescribed by a physiotherapist.

Massage Not just for pleasure or relaxation, this can speed up recovery and reduce discomfort after a hard training session. Massage can help maintain range of motion in joints and reduce mild swelling caused by injury-related inflammation.

Magnesium An essential mineral that plays a role in over 300 processes in the body including in the cardiovascular system and tissue repair.

Maximum heart rate (MHR) The highest number of times the heart can contract (or beat) in one minute. A very approximate figure can be obtained for adults by using the following formula: 220 – current age = MHR. Athletes often exceed this guideline, but only because they have progressively pushed themselves and increased their strength over time.

Mobility The ability of a joint to move freely through a range of motion. Mobility is very important because if you have restricted joint mobility and you start to load that area with weights during exercise, the chances are that you will compound the problem.

Muscular endurance (MSE) The combination of strength and endurance. The ability to perform many repetitions against a given resistance for a prolonged period. In strength training any more than 12 reps is considered MSE.

Negative-resistance training (NRT) Resistance training in which the muscles lengthen while still under tension. Lowering a barbell, bending down and running downhill are all examples. It is felt that this type of training will increase muscle size more quickly than other types of training, but if you only ever do NRT, you won't be training the body to develop usable functional strength.

Obliques The muscles on both sides of the abdomen that rotate and flex the torso. Working these will have no effect on 'love handles', which are fat that sits above, but is not connected to, the obliques.

Origin All muscles are attached to bone or others muscles by tendons or fascia. The end of the muscle which is not moved during a contraction is the origin, with the moving end being called the insertion. Note that some muscles have more than one origin and insertion.

Overtraining Excessive amounts of exercise, intensity, or both volume and intensity of training, resulting in fatigue, illness, injury and/or impaired performance. Overtraining can occur in individual parts of the body or throughout, which is a good reason for keeping records of the training you do so you can see if patterns of injuries relate to a certain time or types of training you do throughout the year.

Patience With strength training – more than any other type of exercise – patience is essential. When you exercise the results are based on the ability of the body to 'change', which includes changes in the nervous system as well as progressive improvements in the soft tissues (muscles, ligaments and tendons). While it is not instantly obvious why patience is so important, it becomes clearer when you consider how, for example, the speed of change differs in the blood rich muscles at a faster rate than the more avascular ligaments and tendons. Improvements take time so be patient.

Pectorals The muscles of the chest, also known as 'the pecs'. Working the pecs will have a positive effect on the appearance of the chest, however, despite claims, it is unlikely that working the pecs will have any effect on the size of female breasts although it can make them feel firmer if the muscle tone beneath them is increased.

Pelvic floor (PF) Five layers of muscle and connective tissue at the base of the torso. The male and female anatomy differs in this area, however, strength and endurance is essential in the PF for both men and women if you are to attain maximum strength in the core. Most of the core training or stability products work the PF.

Periodisation Sums up the difference between a long-term strategy and short-term gains. Periodisation is where you plan to train the body for different outcomes throughout a year or longer. The simplest version of this method would be where a track athlete worked on muscle strength and growth during the winter and then speed and maintenance of muscle endurance during the summer racing season.

Planes of motion The body moves through three planes of motion. Sagittal describes all the forward and back movement; frontal describes the side to side movements; and transverse describes the rotational movements. In everyday life most of the movements we go through involve actions from all three planes all of the time – it is really only 'artificial' techniques, such as biceps curls and deltoid raises, that call upon just one plane at a time.

Plyometrics An explosive movement practised by athletes, for example, two-footed jumps over hurdles. This is not for beginners or those with poor levels of flexibility and/or a limited range of motion.

Prone Lying face down, also the standard description of exercises performed from a lying face down position. The opposite of supine (see below).

Protein A vital nutrient that needs to be consumed every day. Carbohydrates provide your body with energy, while protein helps your muscles to recover and repair more quickly after exercise. Foods high in protein include whey protein, which is a by-product of the dairy industry and is consumed as a shake; fish, chicken, eggs, dairy produce (such as milk, cheese and yoghurt), beef and soya.

Increased activity will increase your protein requirements. A lack of quality protein can result in loss of muscle tissue and tone, a weaker immune system, slower recovery and lack of energy. The protein supplements industry has developed many convenient methods for consuming protein in the form of powders, shakes and food bars, most of which contain the most easily digested and absorbable type of protein, whey protein.

Pyramid A programming method for experienced weight trainers. A set of the same exercises are performed at least three times, each set has progressively fewer repetitions in it, but greater resistance. When you reach the peak of the pyramid (heaviest weight) you then perform the same three sets again in reverse order. For example, going up the pyramid would ask for 15 reps with 10kg, 10 reps with 15kg, 5 reps with 20kg. Going down the pyramid would require 10 reps with 15kg, 15 reps with 10kg.

Quadriceps The groups of muscles at the front of the thighs, also known as 'the quads'. They are usually the first four muscle names that personal trainers learn, but just in case you have forgotten the four are: vastus intermedius, rectus femoris (that's the one that's also a hip flexor), vastus lateralis and vastus medialis.

Range of motion (ROM) The degree of movement that occurs at one of the body's joints. Without physio equipment it is difficult to measure a joint precisely, however, you can easily compare the shoulder, spine, hip, knee and ankle on the left side with the range of motion of the same joints on the right side.

Recoil The elastic characteristic of muscle when 'stretched' to return the body parts back to the start positions after a dynamic movement.

Recovery/rest The period when not exercising and the most important component of any exercise programme. It is only during rest periods that the body adapts to previous training loads and rebuilds itself to be stronger, thereby facilitating improvement. Rest is therefore vitally important for progression.

Repetitions How many of each movement you do, also known as 'reps'. On training programmes you will have seen three numerical figures that you need to understand – reps, sets and circuits.

Repetition max (RM) The maximum load that a muscle or muscle group can lift. Establishing your 1RM can help you select the right amount of weight for different exercises and it is also a good way of monitoring progress.

Resistance training Any type of training with weights, including gym machines, barbells and dumbbells and bodyweight exercises.

Resting heart rate (RHR) The number of contractions (heartbeats) per minute when at rest. The average RHR for an adult is approx 72BPM, but for athletes it can be much lower.

Scapula retraction Not literally 'pulling your shoulders back', but that is a good cue to use to get this desired effect. Many people develop rounded shoulders, which when lifting weights puts them at a disadvantage because the scapular cannot move freely, so by lifting the ribs and squeezing the shoulder blades back the shoulder girdle is placed in a good lifting start position.

Sciatica Layman's term for back pain which radiates through the spine, buttocks and hamstrings. Usually due to pressure on the sciatic nerve being shortened, which runs from the lower back and down the legs, rather than being a problem with the skeleton. Most often present in people who sit a lot. Core training, massage and flexibility exercises can frequently cure the problem.

Set A block of exercises usually put together to work an area of the body to the point of fatigue, so if you were working legs you may do squats, lunges and calf raises straight after each other, then repeat them again for a second 'set'.

SMR – self myofascial release SMR is the general term used to describe most types of manual therapy that is looking to have an effect upon the soft tissue under the skin, e.g. massage with hands, rollers or electronic devices. Gripping and squeezing a muscle, rubbing, kneading or massaging a muscle all count as SMR methods, as does foam rolling – so for clarity all foam rolling exercises are SMR but not all types of SMR are foam rolling.

Speed, agility and quickness (SAQ)® Although in fact a brand name, this has become the term used to describe a style of exercises or drills which are designed to improve speed, agility and quickness. Very athletic and dynamic, often including plyometric movements.

Stretch A balanced approach to stretching is one of the most important elements of feeling good and reducing the likelihood of developing non-trauma soft tissue injuries. When we lift weight clearly the muscle fatigues and as a result at the end of the session the overall muscle (rather than individual fibres) can feel 'tight' or shortened. Doing a stretch will help return the muscle to its pre-exercise state. Dynamic stretching (rhythmic movements to promote optimum range of movement from muscle/joints) should be performed pre-workout.

Superset Similar to a set, but each sequential exercise is performed with no rest in between. The moves in a superset are selected to ensure that they relate to each other, for example, an exercise that focused on shoulders and triceps, such as a shoulder press, would be followed by another shoulder/triceps move, such as dips.

Supine Lying face up, also the standard description of exercises performed from a lying face up position. The opposite of prone (see above).

Tabata® A type of HIIT exercise that has very specific timing, named after its creator, Professor Izumi Tabata. It involves working at extremely high levels of intensity for just 20 seconds followed by an inactive 10 seconds recovery repeated eight times.

Tendon Connective tissue that attaches muscles to bones. Muscle and tendon tissue merge together progressively, rather than there being a clear line where tendon starts and muscle finishes. Like ligaments, a tendon has fewer blood vessels running through it and is less flexible than muscle tissue.

Time As a personal trainer, I have been asked many times, 'What is the best time of day to exercise?' The answer depends. If you are an athlete training almost every day perhaps twice a day, then I would say that strength training in the morning could be more productive than at other times due to the body clock and fluctuating hormone levels throughout the day. However, if the question is asked by a casual exerciser with an average diet and a job and busy lifestyle, my answer would be to exercise at any time of the day, as exercise is a productive use of your valuable free time.

Torsion Stress on the body when external forces twist it about the spinal axis.

Training partner A training partner can be a person who keeps you company and motivates you while you exercise or they can also take the role of being your 'spotter' when you are lifting heavy weights. With foam rolling, certain actions benefit from another person being available to help you stabilise.

Transversus abdominis A relatively thin sheet of muscle which wraps around the torso. This is the muscle that many people think they activate by following the instruction of 'pull your stomach in', however, that movement is more likely to be facilitated by the main abdominals. For your information, a flat stomach is more likely to be achieved by simply standing up straight, as this ensures the correct distance between the ribs and pelvis.

Triceps Muscles at the back of the upper arms. They make up approximately two-thirds of the diameter of the upper arm, so if arm size is your goal, working the triceps will be a priority.

Trigger points Trigger points are hot spots spread around the body where there is a natural tendency for increased amounts of tension or inflammation generally where a selection of muscles attach via a tendon to perform their tasks, they also correspond with many of the known acupressure points. Conservatively there are over 100 potential trigger points around the body and even if you have no understanding of biomechanics and anatomy they are easy to identify with your thumb/finger and some pressure. The easiest to find is where the pectoral major muscle connects to the shoulder: put your finger on your collar bone near your shoulder then move down and slightly back towards the body's centre line where it feels soft then press firmly – ouch! That's a trigger point! Not to be confused with Trigger Point Therapy®, which is a product manufacturer and educational company specialising in foam rolling.

Vertebrae Individual bones that make up the spinal column. The intervertebral discs that sit between them are there to keep the vertebrae separated, cushion the spine and protect the spinal cord.

VO_2 max The highest volume of oxygen a person can infuse into their blood during exercise. A variety of calculations or tests can be used to establish your VO_2 max; these include measuring the heart rate during and after aerobic activity. As each of these tests includes a measurement of the distance covered as well as the heart's reaction to activity, the most popular methods of testing VO_2 max are running, stepping, swimming or cycling for a set time and distance.

Warm-up The first part of any workout session that is intended to prepare the body for the exercise ahead of it. I find it is best to take the lead from the sports world and base the warm-up exactly on the movements you will do in the session. So if you are about to do weights rather than jog, go through some of the movements unloaded to prepare the body for the ranges of motion you will later be doing loaded.

Warm-down The slowing down or controlled recovery period after a workout session. A warm-down can include low level cardio work to return the heart rate to a normal speed as well as stretching and relaxation.

about the author

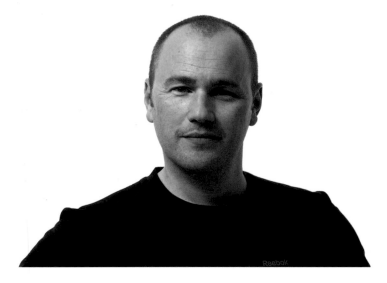

STEVE BARRETT is a former national competitor in athletics, rugby, mountain biking and sport aerobics. His career in the fitness industry as a personal trainer spans over 25 years. His work as a lecturer and presenter has taken him to 42 countries including the United States, Russia and Australia.

For many years Steve delivered Reebok International's fitness strategy and implementation via their training faculty Reebok University. He gained the title and certification of Reebok Global Master Trainer, which is a certification that required a minimum of three years' studying, presenting and researching both practical and academic subjects. In this role between 2000 and 2008 he lectured and presented to more than 20,000 fellow fitness professionals and students. Steve played a key role in the development of the training systems and launch of two significant products in the fitness industry: the Reebok Deck and Reebok Core Board®.

As a personal trainer, in addition to teaching the teachers and working with the rich and famous, he has been involved in the training of many international athletes and sports personalities at Liverpool FC, Arsenal FC, Manchester United FC, the Welsh RFU and UK athletics.

Within the fitness industry he has acted as a consultant to leading brand names, including Nestlé, Kelloggs, Reebok and Adidas.

His media experience includes being a guest expert for the BBC and writing for numerous publications including *The Times*, *The Independent*, *The Daily Telegraph*, *Runner's World*, *Men's Fitness*, *Rugby News*, *Health & Fitness*, *Zest*, *Ultra-FIT*, *Men's Health UK*, *Australia* and many more.

Steve's expertise is in the development of logical, user friendly, safe and effective training programmes. The work that he is most proud of, however, isn't his celebrity projects, but the changes to ordinary people's lives that never get reported.

Now that he has been teaching fitness throughout his 20s, 30s and now 40s, he has developed a tremendous ability to relate to the challenges that people face to incorporate exercise into their lifestyle, and while the fitness industry expects personal trainers to work with clients for a short period of time, Steve has been working with many of his clients for nearly two decades, continuously evolving to meet their changing needs. His fun and direct approach has resulted in many couch potatoes running out of excuses and transforming into fitness converts.

Steve Barrett can be found on Twitter as @GuyInShorts and via his website sodoto.com

index